Heading

Heading South?

The Style Guide For Women Over 40

Forget Gravity! Look and Feel Fabulous
Whatever Your Size or Shape

Sue Donnelly

First Published In Great Britain 2006
by www.BookShaker.com

© Copyright Sue Donnelly

Typeset in Trebuchet

*This book is dedicated to my mum-in-law Audrey who,
in her 80's, is still an inspiration to women of all ages.*

*Thanks also to Sally for suggesting
such a fantastic title.*

Contents

Foreword

If you've ever looked in the mirror and felt a bit, well, disappointed, then looked in your wardrobe and felt there was just nothing in there that would give you the lift you need, it's time to read Sue's latest upbeat book.

Full of wit, and fashion wisdom, it's packed with style tips that not only help you feel more up to date as a 40+ woman in the ever-changing world of the catwalk, but also help you feel more confident, more like the real you.

Because in the end that's what fashion should be all about - finding the unique style that suits you, complements your body shape and your personality. Not about twiglet-thin teenagers prancing down a Milan runway in barely-there drapery no-one sane would ever wear.

If you've lost your fashion va-va-vroom, Sue's the woman to help you get it back - that's why we love her regular column, 'The Fashion Fixer' in Health Plus magazine. Sue's as down-to-earth as you can get, knows all the best tricks, and won't force you to stand in your underwear in front of a TV audience in order to help you find your dream wardrobe.

Phew!

At Health Plus we celebrate real women with real lives who want to look and feel their best every day in their 40s, 50s and beyond. Heading South? captures that same spirit - and we heartily recommend it.

Colette Harris
Editor, Health Plus Magazine

Preface

When I first read "Heading South" I was immediately impressed by its "can do" readable style full of simple, practical ideas and exercises written with great humour and sensitivity.

As an Image Consultant and Life Coach working with women facing extreme self esteem and body image challenges, I found this book an invaluable reference guide. I would have no hesitation in recommending to them as it is tactful, insightful and realistic in its approach. Once these painful issues are addressed women are transformed and liberated.

As a woman rapidly approaching my 50th birthday, and in complete denial about the disappearing years, I laughed out loud - someone has noticed me at last! My neuroses, which I thought were unique, have been put down on paper. What a relief that I'm not alone in the way I think about my body.

'Heading South' is a great reality check. It has helped me realise there are endless possibilities to remain authentically and naturally beautiful in a flexible way where my own image and appearance can evolve creatively. I found it reassuring and uplifting.

This book is a thoroughly good read and I know of so many people who would find this book invaluable -it would make a great gift. Thank you, Sue, for your inspiration in writing this book, which combines imagine consultancy and life coaching effortlessly and seamlessly together – it is so pickup-able and so un put-down able. It really hits the point.

Anna Libby
LifeCoach and Image Consultant
www.liberty-works.co.uk

Skip The Scalpel

*"Please don't retouch my wrinkles.
It took me so long to earn them."*
Anna Magnani - Film Star

I don't know about you, but when I look in the mirror these days it's always a bit of a shock. What's happened to my body? The bags under my eyes could easily hold the weekly supermarket shopping, my bottom is desperately trying to reach my knees and I have a roll of flesh round my middle that would come in handy if I happened to be drowning. I'm also pretty sure I have cellulite, but I'd need to pop my specs on to make absolutely certain!

To project a youthful appearance I could always opt for the miracles of plastic surgery. Unfortunately, having had two non-cosmetic operations in the past, I know that I scar badly so this is a non-starter for me. As they say, "better the devil (or in my case, the body) you know."

I could of course resort to that multi-million pound industry – dieting. Having suffered in my long distant past with eating disorders, I know to my cost that these do not work on a long-term basis.

Some psychologists believe that because the word diet contains the word ''die' the brain is automatically programmed to fight against it. It is far more successful to embark on a 'healthy eating programme' as this is a positive affirmation, which the mind prefers.

I am not saying that cosmetic procedures or weight control are wrong, only that this book will not include them as options. There are plenty of well researched books on these topics if you choose to go that route.

This book is about how to feel good and look great when your body is fighting the laws of gravity.

If, like me, you are around 50 years old then the world should be your oyster. This is the time when we have more freedom, more wealth and more wisdom than in our previous years.

Dwelling on how you used to look isn't helpful when you may still have another 30 years or more to live.

Feeling down about the way you look will drain your confidence and prevent you from living the best life you can. On the other hand, when you look good, you feel good and your self-esteem increases. In turn, this will enable you to project yourself with more conviction and confidence. Others are drawn to you, so you are likely to gain more positive responses from work associates, family, friends and even strangers.

And guess what – your confidence increases even more.

Gone are the days when reaching 50 means elasticated waistbands and tightly permed grey hair.

You only have to look at women these days to know that you can still turn heads even when you are older.

Sharon Stone and Trisha Goddard, both in their late 40's, look fantastic despite having major personal setbacks.

Dawn French and Lorraine Kelly also look fantastic even though neither have model girl figures.

Kim Basinger and Annie Lennox look wonderful for women in their 50's and both have had their share of ups and downs.

Barbara Streisand, 62, is a great example of someone who went against advice and decided to keep her face as nature intended. Her nose gives her a unique beauty which is very compelling.

Diane Keaton's quirkiness and beauty is brought to the fore by her wonderful style and the clothes she wears.

Honor Blackman has recently been seen in magazines and on billboards as the model for M&S, and she's in her 70's.

Katie Boyle and Dame Judi Dench may not have perfect bodies but they still radiate sex appeal in their 8th decade. So it is possible to look sensational even if you're heading south – you just need to know how.

What this book doesn't set out to do is change the intrinsic you. Your "self" is what you are all about.

My aim is to show you how to dress in a way that reflects your inner values, your personality and your body shape. The result – an authentic and confident you.

So if you're on that journey south but it seems more like a Mystery Tour, then do what all sensible travellers do and plan your route. Use this book as your own personal road map, so you can control where you are going and how you get there.

View each chapter as an interesting landmark, which you may or not care to explore. Select what is right for you – at this time – and revisit if necessary. You'll be surprised how pleasant and satisfying your journey, and your ultimate destination, can be.

Enjoy!

Beauty & The Beast

"*I never loved another person the way I loved myself.*"

Mae West - Actress

These days reaching middle age no longer stereotypes us. I have met all sorts of women in their 40's and 50's with completely different lifestyles: small children at home, managing their own companies, hitting the corporate glass ceiling, divorced, widowed, housewives, mature students, empty nesters and so on.

We are all different and that is what is so marvellous about being middle aged NOW.

But sadly, many of us do seem to have something in common. We no longer feel attractive and have lost all sense of how to dress ourselves to look gorgeous.

It would be great if we could have an angel wave a magic wand over us and suddenly 'make' us beautiful.

Sadly, that is not going to happen but that doesn't mean that we too can't be beautiful in our own unique way.

But what is beauty anyway?

It is of course a cliché that "beauty is in the eye of the beholder" or is it?

I carried out a small survey of my own, amongst friends and clients of both sexes and of all age groups. The most important qualities that made a woman beautiful in their eyes were:

- ✓ confidence
- ✓ happiness
- ✓ charisma
- ✓ authenticity

No mention of long blonde hair or big boobs, long legs or flawless skin.

In fact some of the men I spoke to detested the 'plastic' look of someone who had received cosmetic surgery. Interesting.

Unfortunately, most of us dwell on what we lack, rather than the assets we have. Even the most glamorous celebrities bemoan their looks.

Michelle Pfeiffer has said that she looks like a duck, Farrah Fawcett-Majors hates her thick eyelids and Nigella Lawson doesn't like her "sticky-out stomach".

I call these negative thoughts and beliefs 'the beast' and it resides within all of us. We all have parts of our bodies that we don't like and the beast makes sure we won't forget it:

"You can't wear that with your thighs!"

"You look ridiculous in that outfit"

"Look at those wrinkles"

The beast is relentless and we've all had years of its back chat. So much so that we now believe every word it says.

What we forget is that often our 'flaws' are compensated by something which another person would probably kill for.

For instance, if you have a large tum, odds are you'll have a great bum. Large boobs and a short waist usually sit with long legs. Shorter legs often go hand in hand with a long body and a flat tum. A wrinkled face may belong to a slim body whereas a plumper body can often result in younger looking skin.

So turn your attention to the assets you have. Remember, the more you draw attention to your challenges by talking about them, the more others will notice.

So, right now, I would like you to do an exercise for me. I want you to recognise how absolutely gorgeous you are. I know it may be difficult but trust me – you are beautiful in your own right and I need you to know that.

You may want to record the steps of your journey. If so, I would suggest you buy a really beautiful journal which will inspire and motivate you. Any old note book just will not do.

Step 1:

Take a good, long look at yourself in a full length mirror. If you can manage to do this without wearing any clothes then even better.

Step 2:

Let's get the negative stuff out of the way. Write down 10 things you don't like about yourself. I know 10 sounds a lot but I expect the beast will help you along.

Things I don't like about myself:

....

....

....

....

....

....

....

....

....

....

Step 3:

Put a large **X** through every single one of them!

I'm not saying they are unimportant but we don't need to dwell on them – just be aware of their existence. We also need to shut the beast up once and for all and this is a great first step for doing that.

Step 4:

Write down 5 things that you like about yourself.

They don't have to be major things. It could just be that you like your blue eyes, or you have small well-shaped feet. Just be positive about it.

....

....

....

....

....

Step 5:

Now, write down a further 5 things you like about yourself. I know this might be hard but PLEASE do it. Take a really long look at yourself, not a cursory glance. Look at your body as though you had never seen it before. Be curious. What can you discover about yourself?

....

....

....

....

....

See – you ARE gorgeous! Well done!

Step 6:

I want you to imagine that you are falling in love. If you have a partner already then is he or she perfect in the way *they* look? Odds are that they are not but they are still attractive, sexy and fanciable. And so are you.

I want you to look at yourself again. So what if you don't have a "perfect" face – it's what makes you unique. Look at your face and love it. It enables you to smile and laugh.

Imagine you are getting married to yourself. Think about the vows you would make – to love honour and cherish. From now on I would like you to do this for yourself. This means treating yourself as someone special all the time.

Try to see yourself as an entire being, a whole person. I hear so many women saying, "I hate my stomach" or similar remarks on a regular basis. They are so hard on themselves. My Yoga teacher has a saying: "you are not just your yoga mat" and this is the same of ourselves. We are more than just one offending body part. Try to love ALL of yourself in equal measure. Touch your stomach, your thigh, or whatever you don't like and be kind to it. Anoint it with beautiful creams or oils – take care of it like you would a child.

If you receive a compliment about the way you look, I want you to accept it. No more replying with comments like, "this old thing?" or "it only cost..."

Imagine the compliment as a box of your favourite chocolates or a bouquet of flowers. Would you throw them back to the person giving them to you? Of course you wouldn't. But not accepting a compliment is just as rude. You are, in effect, saying that they have no sense of judgment! So practise saying thank you. Nothing more – nothing less – just "thank you" until it feels right.

Step 7:

To keep you motivated, I would like you to think of a positive affirmation about yourself. It must be written with the 3 P's in mind:

✓ Personal

✓ Present Tense

✓ Positive

For instance, you could say, "I'm as gorgeous as a goddess and am treated as such by everyone I meet." or "I'm a sexy siren and men find me captivating." or "I am adored for my beauty, wit and wisdom."

You will need to find something that really resonates with you. It's no good using the word 'sexy' if you don't want to feel that way. Perhaps 'chic and stylish' would be a better fit. It may be that you have to look into the past. Did you feel you were something more special then and now you need to recapture it? Try a few affirmations until you find the one that really captures who you really are deep down.

My Affirmation is:

....

....

....

....

....

Practise saying it out loud to yourself in the mirror.

Write it down and then put it in as many places as you can so you see it on a regular basis. Put it in your purse, on the fridge, in the bathroom mirror and so on. If this is inappropriate, if you share with others for example, then keep it in your handbag or in your underwear drawer but it must be somewhere you visit at least once a day.

Step 8:

Keep noticing how you feel. Has anyone treated you differently? Has the beast gone away yet? Catch yourself in conversation with the beast and tell it how wrong it is. You have no further use for its comments. Step outside yourself and see the beast for what it is – a menace. Make notes in your journal.

Personalise the beast by giving it a name. Mine's called Fred and when we have our conversations, I listen to him and then I say, "Thank you Fred for your input, but those are your opinions, not mine. I am quite capable of making my own mind up!"

If, like me, you have a mind that rarely switches off then it can be more effective to write to your beast instead. If I am feeling particularly low, I write down all the things I think I can't do, for instance, "'I can't wear that dress as my legs are too fat.'" I then go through the letter, cross out all reference to 'I' and change it to, 'Fred says'. When Fred says I can't wear it because my legs are too fat, my immediate reaction is, "'I'll show him!'" and I usually do.

Step 9:

Keep a notebook (or your journal) by your bedside, and every night write down 3 nice things that have happened to you that day. Even if it's a smile and hello from a relative stranger it's worth noting down. You'll go to bed with positive things on your mind and amazingly, you'll feel more positive in the morning too. Watch how these positive feelings increase over the next few weeks in both frequency and power. You'll be amazed.

Step 10:

Read the rest of this book – and apply what you learn.

You have now begun in earnest. This book will show you how to embrace your best qualities and dress them to your advantage, show off your personality and celebrate your uniqueness.

There is only one you and you ARE beautiful!

Sue Donnelly

The Body Beautiful

"A woman's dress should be like a barbed wire fence: serving its purpose without obstructing the view."

Sophia Loren

HOW TO MAKE THE MOST OF YOUR ASSETS

How many times have you spotted a fabulous garment in a shop window and gasped with delight? You've tried it on, bought it and taken it home, but then it remains in the wardrobe because it doesn't look quite right somehow.

I know I've done this countless times.

For me, it's usually when I'm trying to look feminine or when there's a big event coming up like a wedding or a party. The garment in question is usually something floaty and romantic and I ache to look good in it. But I don't.

As with everything, there is a good, scientific reason for this.

Think about Christmas and the time you spend wrapping all those presents. I don't know about you but I'm not too bad when the gift is a book or a box of some sort but as soon as I attempt to wrap something with curved edges I start having problems.

The same problem can also apply to "wrapping" our bodies. Attempting to dress a curvy body in a stiff, starchy fabric is as difficult as wrapping a golf ball in an envelope. It won't fit properly unless lots of adjustments are made.

Even the most expensive paper will not enhance the shape of the object. Furthermore, the package tends to look both bigger and thrown together, however hard you've tried.

Conversely, a straight, angular object like a ruler does not fit well inside a flimsy wrapping. The corners poke through and the wrapping easily slips.

I'm not suggesting any of us is completely rotund or as straight as a stick but all of us lean more towards one shape than the other.

I often see older, larger ladies dressed in a cotton shift dress, usually with a round neck and no sleeves. I believe they wear clothes like these because they think they will hide their bodies but, in actual fact, all they are doing is making themselves look bigger and less shapely.

I remember the surprise and delight of one of my clients with a fuller figure, after we divested her of this type of garment. A gently flared skirt and a jacket with a nipped in waist made her look and feel like a siren. Her figure was back and it was terrific.

Looking at your body in an objective way and understanding your unique shape will help you determine how you can dress it in a way that will always look fantastic.

Looking good and feeling great are inextricably linked. Understanding your assets and being able to capitalise on them will provide you with the means to create your own personal style.

Neither contoured (round) or angular (straight) is the best option in all cases because both can look terrific if you understand some of the style principles that apply to you and use them accordingly.

Step 1:

Take a good look in a full length mirror – preferably in your undies.

- Work from the shoulders and down to your waist area.

- Do your shoulders slope or are they straight?

- Are your upper arms and shoulders softly padded or are they quite bony?

- Is your waist defined with hips that flare?

Turn to the side view:

- Is your bust larger than a D cup?

- Does the small of your back curve in or is it straight?

If you answered yes to the first part of the questions then your upper body is contoured. If you answered yes to the second part then it's angular.

Step 2:

Let's look at your bottom half.

Turn to the front view:

- Do you have definite hips that curve or are they "boyish"?

- Do you have a curve around the saddle bag area or are your legs straight?

Turn again to the side:

- Is your bottom rounded or flattish?

- Do you have a tum?

If you answered yes to the first part of the question then your upper body is contoured. If you answered yes to the second part then it's angular.

It is possible to have a different bodyline for the upper and lower halves of your body.

The line of your body determines the types of fabric that will suit it best. This includes its cut and also the patterns and finishes.

In my case, the flimsy, floaty materials that I tried to wear to look feminine were too lightweight for my angular frame. Bones I didn't even know I had poked through the fabric, the straps kept falling down my shoulders, my bust became non-existent (this is bad news) and I looked, and felt, really uncomfortable. Not how you want to feel when attending an important event.

My attempt to look more romantic revolved around emulating the success of curvier women to achieve this look rather than dressing to enhance my own uniqueness.

Think also of someone like Pamela Anderson. Try and picture her trying to fit into a stiff cotton shirt. She may pull it of because of who she is, but for most of us, it doesn't work. You will look as though you are fighting with your clothes. They won't sit properly, you'll be constantly fiddling with them and you'll appear ill at ease.

So here are some guidelines to help you dress your body so that you'll always look and feel fabulous.

Fabrics:

Rounder bodies (contoured) look best in soft fabrics that drape and skim. The fabric should be able to move with you rather than constrict. It should enhance your curves rather than squash or flatten.

Straighter (angular) bodies suit stiff, starchy fabrics. This applies to all items of clothing including jeans (lycra for contoured bodies).

Patterns:

Patterns and designs look great if they reflect your overall bodyline. Stripes, checks and other geometric shapes enhance the lines of an angular body. Abstract patterns, curves, spots, paisley and florals suit a contoured shape. Everyone can wear plain fabrics. but be aware of texture. Shiny fabrics will enlarge, matt fabrics will slim.

Cut:

The cut of a garment is essential to make the most of your natural shape. Look for straight seams, sharp lapels, slash pockets and straight hems if you are angular. A softer, more rounded cut is better suited to those with curves. Look for rounded lapels, curved seams (or less structure if you're larger), rounded hems and pockets with flaps.

SIZE IS EVERYTHING

They say size isn't important but in fact, where style is concerned, it is. The patterns you wear, the weight of the fabric, your accessories, even your heel height will look considerably better if the size reflects that of your body. If you fail to choose clothing that fits your scale then you're in danger of looking eccentric, over-powering or lost.

Think about Dame Edna Everage. Probably not an icon you'd wish to emulate but she does demonstrates the point. Everything she wears, from her over sized specs, to the glittery costumes and the "big" hair yell bad taste. But some of us do this on a regular basis without even being aware of it.

Look at the diagram below:

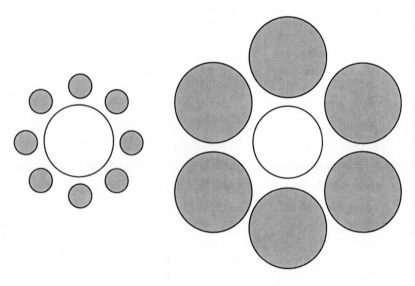

Which of the inner circles looks smaller?

Actually the circles are the same size. The one surrounded by the larger circles only appears to be smaller because it is overshadowed by the larger ones.

If you wear clothes or patterns that are too large for you, you will appear swamped. Unfortunately, you will not look smaller, just lost, so if you're larger than you'd like to be then wearing oversized clothes is not an easy alternative to exercise or eating sensibly!

Conversely, if you wear too small a scale, you will look much bigger. Can't believe many of us would want that!

While on the subject of size, please don't get fixated with the size label in your garments because there is no standardisation of sizing in UK female clothing. Even in the same store, you will often find a size 10 that's bigger than a size 12.

So, if the label upsets you – cut it out and throw it away.

You'll be pleased to know that scale is relative to bone structure and not to the amount of fat you carry. So ladies, when I ask you to find a tape measure, hopefully, you'll not have a heart attack.

Step 1:

Take the tape measure and measure around your wrist.

If your wrist measures:

- Under 51/2 inches/ 14 cm – you're small scale
- 51/2 – 61/2 inches/ 14-16cm – medium
- Over 61/2/ 16cm – large

Height is also a consideration but it is possible to be a tall person (over 5ft6") and have a small scale or be short (under5ft3") and have large scale.

I previously mentioned my longing to look feminine and how the fabric of my floaty outfit didn't suit my angular body. There was also another reason why it didn't look great; the scale was wrong.

As someone who is medium to large scale, the weight of the chiffon was too light. To address this problem, all I needed to do was wear something thicker underneath. Hey presto, problem solved!

To get an idea of scale worn badly, imagine a large scale lady spilling over the edge of her small, kitten heels or a tiny lady wearing huge platform shoes.

Get the idea?

So here are some guidelines for you to think about:

Small scale:

- Fabric weights should be light.

- Patterns should be small and also reflect your bodyline.

- Accessories (apart from specs which are covered in a later chapter) should reflect both your scale and your bodyline. A small, floppy handbag will look fantastic on a small scale contoured woman.

- Shoes should have a small, neat heel.

Medium scale:

- Fabric should be of medium weight.

- Patterns should be medium size and reflect your bodyline.

- Accessories (apart from specs which are covered in a later chapter) should reflect both your scale and your bodyline. A medium size, stiff leather handbag will look fantastic on a medium scale angular woman. If you're contoured, opt for a fabric that moves, such as suede or fabric.

- Shoes should have a medium heel. If you want to add drama, you can choose stiletto or platform as long as the rest of your outfit is in scale.

Large scale:

- Fabrics should be the heaviest weights.

- Patterns should be large and also reflect your bodyline.

- Accessories (apart from specs which are covered in a later chapter) should reflect both your scale and your bodyline. A large handbag will look fantastic on a large scale woman. Choose stiff leather if you're angular and a softer leather if you're contoured.

- Shoes should have a chunky heel. If you wish, you can go for height. It all depends on how tall you want to look.

I remember one of my wardrobe weeding sessions with a client who had a small to medium frame. She showed me her brand new coat which was patterned with very large roses over the entire garment. I was very keen to let it go but she was adamant it was staying. In the end, I donned the coat myself and asked her for her opinion. She burst out laughing and said that I looked like a garden trellis! We had no problem disposing of the awful garment after that. However, to be fair to the coat, it would have looked fantastic worn correctly on someone with a larger scale.

The texture of a fabric is also important. A shiny fabric will make you look larger than a matt one. Just think of a man with a beer belly in a football shirt and you'll know what I mean.

So use matt fabrics if you don't want to attract attention to a certain part of your body. This also applies to light and dark colours. A dark colour will make you look slimmer than a lighter one. So beware of wearing light, shiny fabrics on areas that you're not comfortable with.

On the whole, a textured garment will create a softer outline than one with sharp tailoring. If you have an angular body then you are better off steering clear of loose, nubby type fabrics. Stick to fabrics that are tightly woven like gabardine or twill. If you are very curvy, texture can add bulk to your frame, so choose fabrics that fall in soft folds such as jersey, wool crepe and wool/silk blends.

My scale is

....

Fabric weight is

....

Patterns are

....

....

Accessories

....

....

....

Drama can be created by up-scaling. A large piece of jewellery (including a watch), a higher heel, or a bolder pattern can all get you noticed. Just choose ONE area only or you'll end up looking like Dame Edna.

We want drama not pantomime!

To be truly authentic in the way you dress, you will need to 'imitate' your features within your clothing. If you have freckled skin, for instance, you will look great in a textured, multi-coloured scarf. If you have thick hair, opt for thickness in one of your fabrics. If you have smooth skin, you'll look better in smooth, satiny materials.

Repeat your eye colour in your garments or your accessories for that added je ne sais quoi.

As we get older, our hair turns greyer and our lines become more pronounced. This means we can open up to new possibilities in our clothing. The once smooth fabrics might now give way to textured or patterned.

Grey hair could look absolutely fabulous matched with a long grey evening dress and silver accessories. The important thing is to make changes that reflect the change in you.

A word about quality. In the past, it was always the unwritten rule that you should buy the best quality fabrics you could afford when purchasing your clothes. These days, it seems that people are in two camps: those who buy designer labels and bespoke tailoring and those who prefer the "throw away" culture of cheaper items.

With top names designing for high street stores (Jasper Conran and Ben De Lisi for Debenhams, Karl Lagerfeld and Stella McCartney for H&M) you can now achieve a stylish look at a great price.

Even well known fashionistas such as Naomi Campbell are pairing luxury designer garments with those from chain stores on the High Street.

The let down is always with the accessories. Unless you're looking for a "fun" look, choose accessories that are classic and show quality and good taste. At important meetings, for instance, you can bet money on the fact that your shoes, bag, watch and jewellery will be noticed.

Remember – fit is everything. You can spend thousands of pounds on designer labels but if they don't fit you properly, don't make the most of your body shape, or aren't appropriate for your lifestyle then they are destined for the charity shop before you've even got them home.

I always spend my money on one great handbag per year. This year it was a tote made from soft, green leather and it really does make a statement. I coveted the bag for 6 weeks before actually spending my hard earned cash. I have never regretted the decision to purchase. Not only does it look fantastic – I get lots of admiring comments from people I meet – but it has been designed well. Lots of places to hold my mobile, books, files and all the paraphernalia I need for my everyday life. Whenever I put the bag on my shoulder I feel a great sense of joy. As this is a daily occurrence, I feel wonderful on a regular basis.

If you can't decide whether a garment or an accessory is really worth what you're paying for it, ask yourself, "Does it have the wow factor?" If it doesn't, leave it because you're bound to find something you'll like better just around the corner.

It's All An Illusion

"My legs aren't so beautiful. I just know what to do with them."

Marlene Dietrich - Actress

THE ART OF CHEATING

Whether or not we buy quality clothing, most of us no longer look like the models and celebrities we see in magazines. However - all is not lost. I'm not able to airbrush you, but I can show you how to cheat so you'll certainly look more model-like than you did before.

Apart from being beautiful, models have something else - Perfect Proportions:

- Shoulders wider than hips

- Long waist

- Long legs

As long as we can create the illusion of having these proportions in our own bodies, we too can look like we belong on the cat walk.

Coco Chanel once said, "Fashion is architecture – it is a matter of proportions." She's right. It's all about lines. Those of you with an interest in art, architecture or maybe geometry will know there are 4 types:

1. Vertical – runs up and down.

2. Horizontal – runs side to side.

3. Diverging/Converging – creates a V. Diverging at the widest points, converging where they meet at the narrowest point.

4. Diagonal – from top to bottom, left to right or vice versa.

Our natural shape can be altered by using these lines so a different image is perceived by the viewer:

- Vertical lines create length.

- Horizontal and diverging lines create width.

- Converging lines will narrow.

- The effect of diagonal lines depends on the angle. The more vertical, the more length is created, the more horizontal, the more shortening.

Clever use of lines can make short legs appear longer, small busts look larger, shoulders look wider and so on.

The first thing to do is to understand your own proportions. Just because you have to purchase longer length trousers does not necessarily mean you have long legs, only that you are tall.

When we measure proportion we are looking at the ratio of one part of the body to another – in this case the legs versus the torso and head and the hips in relation to the shoulders.

Step 1:

Let's start with the waist, as this is the easiest one to look at. It's not the measurement around the girth but the length between your breastbone and your waist that is important.

Place the flat of your hand underneath your bustline.

Then place the other hand underneath the first. If both fit easily between your waist indent and your breastbone, you are long waisted. If the second hand doesn't easily fit, you are short waisted

Generally speaking – if you are long waisted then you will have short legs and if you are long legged you'll typically have short legs. This principle often applies to naturally large breasted women too, who tend to be short waisted and long legged.

Lucky you – large boobs and long legs!

Step 2:

This step is optional as it's quite difficult to do on your own. If you have already discovered that your waist is long or short then you can assume that your legs are the opposite. However, if you want to check you can do the following exercise...

Take off your shoes. Stand against a wall (for balance) and bend one leg at 90 degrees to your body. Ask a friend to take a tape measure and measure the distance from where the crease occurs at the top of the bent leg to the floor – in other words – your inside leg measurement. Now measure from the same crease to the top of your head. If the first measurement is smaller then you have short legs in proportion to your height. If it's longer then you have long legs.

Step 3:

Shoulders: Stand in front of a mirror and check whether the edges of your shoulders are wider or narrower than your hips at the widest point. If you're unsure then ask a friend to check from the back view.

My proportions are

1. Legs ....

2. Waist ....

3. Shoulders ....

I am one of those people, who at 5ft4", have a very long body and really short legs. Delegates at my workshops are amazed when I impart this fact. They believe I am taller than my actual height and have legs that go on forever.

I use my knowledge to change what I haven't got naturally into something I'd love to have. Who cares if it's cheating?

Here's how it can work for you...

Short Legs/Long Waist:

Need vertical lines to create length.

The general principle here is short – shorter length jackets, shorter length tops and shorter length skirts.

The longest jackets to suit you will just cover the cheeks of your bottom. Any longer and your legs will shorten. Skirt hems should sit around knee length.

- Avoid turn ups on trousers as the horizontal line will shorten the leg. And definitely avoid any trousers with tapered legs. Make sure they are long enough. They should touch where your toes crease. If you are petite then you can afford to have trousers trailing on the ground.

- Boot leg cut is very flattering for shorter legs.

- Vertical stripes or a centre crease give the illusion of length.

- Shorter skirts (knee length) are more flattering than long ones. Wear with knee high boots that touch the hem of the skirt or coordinating tights. Any gap will shorten the leg. Asymmetric hems are also a good idea.

- Pointed toe shoes will lengthen, rounded will shorten as will any horizontal bars in the design. Avoid ankle straps at all costs, especially if calves are thick. Try flip–flop V design rather than sliders in the summer.

- Heels make legs look longer.

- Jackets should be no longer than bum length. Shorter jackets look good as long as you have no challenges round the hip or tum area.

- Belts should match bottoms rather than tops.

Long Legs/Short Waist:

Needs vertical lines to create length.

The general principle here is long – longer jackets, longer tops and longer skirts. The shortest jacket length should just cover the cheeks of your bottom. If you wear a shorter jacket, your waist will also shorten and you will look out of proportion.

- Avoid any horizontal lines on your top half as they will widen and make you look fatter. Vertical lines will slim.

- Drop waisted or hipster trousers give length to your upper body.

- Single-breasted jackets and cardigans flatter whilst double breasted will give the illusion of width. Keep the jacket open if you want to appear slimmer.

- Empire line dresses and tops will give the illusion of length in the torso, as will tops with an asymmetric hemline.

- Try trousers and skirts without waistbands.

- If you do wear a belt then match it to your top half not the bottom

- Wear shirts and tops worn out rather than tucked in.

- Longer skirts and jacket lengths look good.

- Simple unstructured clothing rather than fitted will look better on you.

Narrow shoulders:

Need horizontal or diverging lines to create width.

- Wide lapels and shirt collars give the illusion of width.

- Avoid halter necks as all eyes will be on your boobs! Also avoid raglan, three quarter, or sleeveless garments.

- Try Trench Coats with detail on the shoulder.

- Sleeves with widening lines such as capped, petal, dolman or ruched.

- Off the shoulder styles look good or try wrapping a scarf or pashmina round your shoulders.

- Wear shoulder pads as long as they are fashionable or part of your suit's tailoring.

- Avoid excessive pleating or bulk around the hips as this will also make your shoulders look out of proportion.

- The use of colour can also help distract. Wear darker colours on your bottom half to make the hips look smaller and your shoulders wider. Bright or light colours in shiny fabrics will draw attention whilst dark colours in a matt fabric will deflect.

FIGURE CHALLENGES

Now we've all got long legs, wide shoulders and newly acquired model looks, what else could we wish for?

I know from experience, my own and my clients', that we often have a problem with a certain area of our body. So much so, that we often fixate on it – even though other people rarely notice or cannot understand what we're worried about. If it's real for you though then it won't make much difference what others say – it will still cause you concern.

I have a very low slung bum due to my very long back. From the front I look okay but from the back I always feel my bum is drooping further and further towards my knees. You may not notice this but I do – and that's what counts.

I've now developed a look that completely hides my bum, still gives me a great outline and always looks stylish. A fitted jacket, with a knee length hem, can be worn over jeans, trousers and a skirt. As long as I team it with heels, so I remain in proportion, you cannot tell where my bum is and the rest of my body looks great. This type of jacket also works well to disguise saddle bags. Wearing a wrap cardigan and tying a large bow at the back also takes the attention away from my bum.

It's a question of finding out what works for you and using it to your advantage.

If you have no problems with any part of your body then you can skip the rest of this chapter and move onto the next one. If, like most of us, gravity is taking its toll then keep reading!

Disguising a full bust:

- Women with large boobs often have a short neck. An opening at the neck, such as a V neck or a scoop, will break up the area. Try open neck shirts (the stand up collar will flatter the face), or a crossover V sweater. A closed neckline, for instance a polo neck or a poncho, will make the bust appear larger.

- A full bust means a contoured outline, so stick to curved lines on top. Avoid details and prints that draw focus to the breasts, especially horizontal stripes or pockets.

- The correct bra is essential. It can take pounds off you. Don't wear lacy bras with T-shirts or close fitting fabrics.

- Dark colours in a matt fabric will draw attention from the bust area. Bright colours and shiny fabrics attract attention.

- Longer line jackets, with single breasted fastenings and long sleeves look great on large busts. Try wearing a scarf draped round the neck and falling over the chest area to create length.

- Ruching is great as you can't tell what is you and what is fabric so it hides a multitude of sins.

- Avoid halter neck tops, especially with unsupported boobs and sleeves ending at the bust line.

Enhancing a small bust:

Padded bras and "chicken fillets" are a must if you want to look like you have a cleavage. Aim for a smooth finish under clingier fabrics. Most stores sell seamless T-shirt bras which do the job well.

- Wearing lots of thin layers can add bulk to the chest area without making you look fat.

- Ruching is good as you can't tell between bust size and fabric.

- Pockets, stripes and patterns enhance the chest.

- Short sleeves ending at the bust line create a horizontal line creating width.

- Off the shoulder, halter neck, patterns and textures look great on a smaller chest.

- Light colours in shiny fabrics attract attention.

- Avoid necklines that are too low and going braless.

Hiding a full tum:

To skim is to slim so dress to divert attention away from your mid section.

- Single breasted jackets and coats will lengthen and slim the body, especially if they are longer length.

- Wear the same colour on upper and lower body.

- Try dresses and tops with an empire line or no visible waistline.

- Avoid belts round the waist or things tucked in.

Disguising a pear shaped figure:

The focus needs to be drawn away from the bum and hips.

- Wear long jackets that don't cut across the hip line or your widest point.

- Dark colours on the bottom and lighter colours on your upper body will draw the attention away from your lower half.

- Jewellery and scarves are good diversionary tactics.

- Boot cut trousers/jeans, trousers without waistbands, and drapey fabrics that don't cling are a wise choice.

- Avoid too much detail around the waist such as belt loops or pleating.

BUILD A SECURE FOUNDATION

The wrong underwear can ruin an outfit instantly. Spend time and money on selecting the right size and style. It can instantly transform your shape and make you appear to be pounds lighter. Bras in lacy fabrics worn under a T-shirt or a sheer blouse add lots of bulk so make sure you choose the correct style for your outfit.

If you have large breasts then it is essential that you have yourself measured correctly – probably every 6 months. Manufacturers' sizings can differ widely so don't think because you are a 36D in one bra that you are a 36D in another. Department stores can have up to 40 suppliers for their lingerie, so sizing is bound to differ.

Bras that fit badly not only look horrendous, especially if flesh is spilling out under the cups, but can also lead to sagging of the breast tissue and stretch marks. If that wasn't enough, the wrong size bra can cause headaches, cysts, neck ache and back ache.

The average size of a woman's breast has increased over the years to an E/F cup. As a result, you'll find a much wider selection in larger cup sizes than in previous years. Rigby and Peller (www.rigbyandpeller.com) and Bravissimo (www.bravissimo.com) offer bra's that are sexy even in very large sizes.

The Bottom Line

VPL (visible panty lines) are a real no-no. Larger tums or bums can benefit from knickers that "hold you in." whereas shorts are useful for those with pert behinds. Bridget Jones' "big pants" are definitely out!

Tummy Trouble

A higher waistline coupled with strong fibres are what you need to combat problems in the tummy region. Most department stores have their own ranges in stock. Try them out until you find the one that suits your figure best.

Droopy Drawers

Those of us with very long bodies may find our bottom is a little too close to our knees from the rear view. If so, try Shape Up Briefs by Levante (01277 232301), Falke's Contour Panty (020 7493 8442) or Magic Slimshort which flatten your stomach at the same time (www.figleaves.com).

Thongs

Apparently the thong is now passé. To replace it, you can find seam free, invisible-line knickers called shorts. They won't show through the tightest of skirts or over the top of low cut trousers. You can find similar items at most large department stores and lingerie shops.

Cellulite

To rid yourself of orange peel cheeks or thighs, try www.tightsplease.co.uk. Spanx Original Footless Tights should also do the trick. Playtex also do a range that include a thigh and tummy slimmer (0500 362430).

For that extra special silk dress, knock-em-dead moment, go to Rigby and Peller (www.rigbyandpeller.com). They make an elasticated full body corset that gives freedom and control, so you can relax and enjoy all that lovely attention.

John Lewis is now offering a specially tailored service for control underwear. You can book an appointment, which is free, with your local store's lingerie department.

Stocking Fillers

There's nothing worse than seeing a pair of lily-white, goose-bumpy legs so that's why it's a pleasure to see so many different styles of hose around.

If you're like me and wear tights most of the time (a pair of hold-ups slid down my legs in the middle of a very important presentation I was giving – so never again!) you may find them tight and restrictive around the waist area. Well, problem solved. River Island now stock a variety of tights with a low rise. Hipster Tights start at £4.99 and are available in a wide range of colours and styles.

Woolly or ribbed tights are lovely and warm to wear. They may not seem sexy but can be made to look chic if teamed with a pair of high wedges or some sexy boots.

Crocheted tights can be flattering if made from soft, fine wool. Choose subtlety over loud designs.

Patterned tights. The larger the pattern the less flattering to your legs. Never wear with a printed garment. Patterned tights are best worn with plain clothes. Vertical stripes can lengthen the legs so are useful to the short legged amongst us.

Colourful tights can be wonderful or ghastly. If you're young at heart, brave or both you could try mixing colours that clash such as orange and pink. For the rest of us, match your tights to your skirt and shoes but be slightly daring with the colour you choose. Why not try olive green or deep purple? Make sure they are matt/opaque not shiny as the latter will make your legs look bigger.

Of course, these suggestions may not be the best thing to wear if you're expecting a night of passion but they *will* get you noticed and for all the right reasons!

Here Comes The Sun

---

*"Elegance is good taste,
plus a dash of daring."*

Carmel Snow, Fashion Journalist

Summer is no longer just confined to a couple of months a year. With holidays abroad costing so little these days we can spend as much time in the sun as our bank accounts allow. How do you feel about exposing your flesh to the scrutiny of other holidaymakers? If the answer is, "I hate it!" then take heed of the following advice.

There is swimwear to suit all shapes and sizes. It's just a question of knowing what will make you look even more gorgeous than you already are.

Here are my tips to help enhance your best features and disguise those that you don't like as much.

Large hips:

- If you have large hips or saddlebags along with a smallish bust then opt for a two piece rather than a swimsuit. Small bikini bottoms, especially those with string ties at the side, will elongate legs. Halter necks and ruched tops will create a more balanced bustline. Bikini bottoms with a V-cut waist-band will also work. Bandeau tops look great if they are cinched in the middle rather than going straight across the chest area.

- Many bikinis have different patterns/colours top and bottom so make the most of the new trend. Dark colours on your bottom half will make it look slimmer, while a bright or light colour up top will divert attention away from the hip area.

- If you really don't feel comfortable in a bikini then buy a one piece with high cut legs or try a tankini with a smaller bottom. If you have a large bottom then don't have high waisted bottoms or those that completely cover all of your cheeks. It will look matronly.

- A sarong wrapped loosely round the waist and a large sunhat to balance, completes the look. Carry a bright patterned beach bag over your shoulder to also divert attention away from your hips and balance out your body.

Large tum:

- A one-piece swimsuit is the best bet. If you can find one with ruching down the centre, even better, as the wrinkles disguise any flesh in the folds of the fabric.

- Depending on your overall size, you can use a pattern to detract the eye from the offending area.

- If you have large boobs then you will need a swimsuit that has a lowish neck or your bust can appear "shelf-like" and even more obvious.

- A swimsuit with a medium high cut leg will make the most of longer legs and detract attention away from your middle.

- To cover up, try a V-neck kaftan and a big pair of sun glasses.

Large boobs:

- Avoid halter or high necklines as they will make your bust look enormous. Tops should have support under the bust but make sure it is stylish. You don't want to look like your grandma. A keyhole top can be surprisingly effective, and it's glamorous.

- A sarong tied around the waist is your best cover up option. If you tie it higher on the body or with a halter twist around the neck, it will attract attention to your bust.

Angular:

- A halter neck top will widen shoulders and boobs will appear to be larger. If you are long bodied, try a tankini, as it may feel more comfortable. You can wear athletic looking swimwear, so try racing backs. Beware of triangle tops, as they can flatten your breasts if not padded. Bandeau tops, in a textured or detailed fabric can flatter and add inches, as can strategically placed 'chicken fillets'.

- If you want to look curvier then opt for a swimsuit with keyholes cut out of the sides. Boy shorts can work if you have long legs. If your legs are short then avoid wearing shorts at all costs as you'll look stumpy.

- A pair of linen draw-string trousers look great on this shape. Try a baseball cap, a bandanna or a small bucket hat as your finishing accessory. Alternatively, try a sarong tied around the bust.

Curvy:

- Keep it simple. Block colours look best as they elongate your frame. Choose underwired bra tops, whether in a bikini or a swimsuit, as droopy boobs are not a good look to have. A belted one piece looks great if you have a tiny waist.

- A sarong, a large hat and huge sun glasses will give you film star appeal. Avoid a kaftan as it will hide your curves.

Think about your scale and your complexion. Too large a pattern on a petite frame can swamp and too small on a large frame can add pounds. Black can be slimming, on the right colouring. If you are naturally fair haired, and don't tan well then black may be overpowering. Try brown or blue instead.

Size and fit is critical. Never purchase swimwear if you have to keep adjusting the legs or it's too short in the body. Persevere. The perfect garment awaits you.

Shoes with a wedge or thick sole, coupled with a V frontage such as a flip-flop, will lengthen the legs. Sliders, or any sandal with a horizontal bar, will shorten.

Unless you have a bright complexion (see It's Not All Black and White) steer clear of very bright or garish colours until you have your tan. Stick to muted, neutral tones so you don't look washed out.

Bring out the film star in you. Buy some super sunglasses, add a cocktail (or two) and act as if you are the belle of the beach.

Relax in the knowledge that you look terrific!

It's Not Always Black or White

"Pink is not a colour, it's a state of mind."

Unknown

If I had a pound for every woman I saw wearing black on a regular basis, I'd be a millionaire by now. As we get older, and often larger, we look to black as our safe option. We think it makes us look smaller and more sophisticated.

In fact 70% of women's clothes sold annually in the UK are black. If you are one of the many women who doesn't really suit black then you may be making yourself look tired and drawn instead of slim and chic.

Hundreds of years ago, man did not have names for all the colours we have today. Modern technology has produced a myriad of new shades for us to delight in. One way of labelling that has been with us from the start is that of a warm shade (yellow based) and a cool one (blue based). They were also aware of terms such as dark and light, bright and soft.

These characteristics are what we base our colour analysis on today. By using specific coloured drapes, we can pick out colours that share the same characteristics as your complexion, thus making you look wonderful when you wear them.

It's quite difficult to work out which colours suit you best in a book. So it is far better to have a professional consultation with an image coach if you want to get it absolutely right.

I have defined particular groups below to help you. You may belong to one or more of them depending on your own personal make-up. Use them as a guideline to ascertain what will definitely work for you.

Take it from me that it even works when you're not feeling too well. Clients who wear their most flattering colours have reported that they have been told how marvellous they look even when suffering from a hangover!

UNDERSTANDING YOUR CHARACTERISTICS

- Generally speaking if you are dark haired, dark eyed with a dark skin or one that tans well, you will wear dark colours well.

- Conversely, if you are fair–haired, with a paler skin and hair colour, you will better suit lighter colours.

- If you have red hair and freckles, or olive skin and green eyes, you will have a warm complexion so yellow–based colours will best suit you.

- If you have a pink tone to your skin, blue eyes with ash–blonde or grey hair then you'll have a cool complexion and blue–based colours will look great on you.

- If you have a high contrast between hair and skin (black hair and very pale skin) or your eyes are very bright, you wear bright colours well.

- If there is little contrast between hair, eyes and skin you are muted and suit softer colours.

There are 4 main types, or 'seasons,' which I've detailed as follows:

WINTER Dark, Cool & Bright	AUTUMN Dark, Muted & Warm	SUMMER Light, Cool & Muted	SPRING Light, Bright & Warm
Dark or grey hair

Bright blue, hazel, brown or black eyes

Skin can be fair to very dark. It may have a high contrast to the hair

Look of high contrast or strength | Golden blonde, auburn or brown hair

Soft shades of green, hazel or brown eyes

Skin tone is soft, similar to eye colour with no real contrast and will have a sun kissed look or freckles

Look of warmth or richness | Light to medium ash blonde, mousy or cool light red hair

Pale blue, grey, green or hazel eyes

Blue under-tones to the skin show in a pinkiness which can be fair or medium

Look of delicateness or, English rose | Golden blonde or warm light brunette/ red hair

Bright shades of blue, green, hazel and brown

Yellow undertones show as a sun kissed look on the skin, which will be fair.

Look of lightness, and brightness |

If you're unsure which box you fit into then use the guidelines for your dominant characteristic instead; if you know you are very dark then stick mainly to darker colours and accent with others.

If you do fit into a type shown above then it may be helpful to think about the colours you will find during each of the seasons, as these will be the ones that best suit you:

- **Winter:** Bold, dramatic landscapes, with white snow, black leafless trees, grey skies, deep red berries. This palette includes the bright, deep primary colours, except yellow, and the icy tones of very pale blue, green, pink, violet and white. You can wear suiting in black and charcoal well.

- **Autumn:** Trees with leaves of all shades of gold, orange, green, yellow, red and brown give a good insight into the colours which suit this complexion. They are soft shades and not bright. Cream is a better choice than white. You will look better in chocolate brown or navy suiting. Olive green looks especially good.

- **Summer:** Soft shades of pink, lavender, blue and lemon. All pastels look good on this complexion. Imagine the sun has faded and the colours of the flowers in bloom are no longer bright but have muted tones. Off white is more suitable than a bright white. You will suit grey and a soft navy rather than black in tailored garments.

- **Spring:** Flowers are emerging such as daffodils, and crocuses. Bright shades that have a yellowish tinge but are light rather than dark. Corals, light green and turquoise fit nicely into this palette. Ivory is a better choice than white, which is too cool. You will look good in pale linen colours, beige or brown, rather than black.

Remember, that these guidelines apply to colours worn around your face. If you love a colour and you know it doesn't suit you then wear it somewhere else. I have a fantastic bright green bag. It cost a fortune and I love it but I rarely wear green against my face.

Jewellery, shoes, a watch, a hair ornament or a belt can all pick up aspects of a colour that may be overwhelming if worn head to toe. A lipstick or a coloured mascara or eye pencil will have the same effect.

Another option is to buy patterned or multi coloured garments. As long as the overall colours suit you, a splash of another shade will not hurt.

It is important that you take your personality into account when you wear your colours too. If you are shy then bright colours can propel you into an unwelcome limelight. We see bright colours first, due to their longer wavelengths, so try muted shades instead.

If you are bright, bold or dynamic then you will probably look best in blocks of colour such as black trousers and white top. If you are softer or more gentle then try wearing the same colour in different hues such as a pale olive top with darker olive skirt and a brown belt.

HAIR TODAY GONE TOMORROW

Be wary of hairdressers and makeup ladies who don't understand the difference between cool and warm.

The current trend is for us to be "warmed up". Cosmetic counters offer bronzing powders and fake tans to turn us into bronzed beauties. Hairdressers often promote gold or copper highlights to provide a warm glow around our face. But "being warmed up" doesn't actually suit all of us. In fact we can be in danger of looking jaundiced or sallow with colours that are too yellow for our natural complexion. And I'm guessing that no-one would choose to look ill!

This also can apply to fake tans. Although safer than lying in the sun, the golden look may not suit a naturally pale, cool skin. If you fall into this category then be brave and show off your natural pallor. It works for Madonna.

If you have a cool skin tone then look at shades of plum hair colour rather than auburn; ash-blonde rather than golden blonde. If you have naturally fair hair then keep it fair and don't be tempted to go darker. Unfortunately, pigment does fade as we get older so if your hair was naturally jet black (or very dark) it probably isn't now. Dying it back to its original shade will do you no favours. It will look dyed and probably make you look older.

Either have highlights or opt for a colour about two shades lighter than your original if you want to keep looking youthful.

Highlights can add a natural movement and shine to your hair and are a safer bet than an all over colour. If you are grey then make the most of it by choosing a style that really shows off your crowning glory.

For years I was a golden blonde. I never felt it was quite right but the hairdresser said it suited me and I went along with it. I applied stacks of makeup, bronzers and a really dark lipstick to balance out my look. Now I realise my instinct was correct. I am now a striking silver blonde. As it suits my colouring, I need less makeup, my eyes are brighter and I look younger than I did before. That's the magic of colour!

DRESSING TO CHANGE YOUR APPROACH

There are times in our lives when we can become anxious or nervous. It might be a presentation to the board, an interview, a blind date, meeting your daughter's boyfriend for the first time and so on. We could all do with a little help on these occasions – without hitting the gin bottle.

You may not be aware of it but colour is a powerful medium when it comes to tackling everyday situations.

You may even be wearing a colour which sends outs a signal, albeit subconsciously. Pink, for instance, is thought to be the colour of love, so wearing it may be an attempt to surround ourselves with love or even attract love into our lives. I've seen many of my recently divorced clients wearing pink, even though they may have never worn it beforehand.

Think about situations that might cause anxiety in your life, or occasions when you need to be motivated or inspired.

Using the following guide, discover how wearing a particular colour can help and assist you when you most need it. The colour does not have to apply to the entire outfit, sometimes just a splash will do the trick.

RED: Red has the longest wavelength, so we see it first (think traffic lights, brake lights and so on). It is stimulating and courageous. Wear it if you want to be noticed, powerful, assertive or strong. Politicians often wear a red tie when they have something important to say. The red imitates the colouring in the lips so you will automatically look at the mouth.

ORANGE: A mixture of yellow and red symbolising passion, abundance and fun. Beware though – unless you are deeply tanned not many of us carry off this colour well. So wear as a complimentary or accent colour unless you want to be Tango'd!

YELLOW: An emotional colour that governs extraversion, friendliness, creativity and optimism. It represents our personal power and how we feel about ourselves. A spot of yellow can go a long way to making you feel more confident. This colour looks better on those of us with darker skins, so be careful not to over do it.

GREEN: The least widely worn colour in the UK, perhaps because of its "unlucky" connotations. Green signifies balance, compassion and understanding. A useful colour to wear if you have a difficult client, a confrontation or an apology to make! It's also useful to enable balance within if you feel "out of sorts." Bright lime green suits very few people and can reflect back onto the face giving a green shadow around the jaw. So, unless you want to look like an alien, choose a darker or softer alternative.

BLUE: Governs speech, communication, creative expression and intellect. Wear it when presenting a speech or if you need a clear thought pattern. A serene and soothing colour - it mentally calms. Interestingly, Tony Blair and George W Bush both wore dark navy suits during the Iraq crisis. The message? "Trust us, we know what we are doing." Blue can give you an air of authority.

PURPLE: A spiritual colour which is also thought to represent authenticity, truth and luxury (Cadbury's Dairy Milk was perceived to be very expensive chocolate due to its purple wrapper). It has many links with royalty and the church due to its expensive price years ago.

PINK: Love and femininity. A soothing colour that radiates warmth and love. If you have a warm skin then choose coral instead of pink.

BROWN: Earthy and reliable, though it can be construed as dull. Brown is warmer and softer than black and can look more flattering on warmer skins. Stick to darker shades for maximum impact. Wear if you want to elicit trust and openness.

BLACK: Everyone's favourite 'safe' bet. Exudes sophistication, glamour, efficiency, authority and security. Often worn as a slimming aid (though this does not work for everyone) it can drain and become serious. Wear with caution unless you know it suits you.

WHITE: White is a total reflection and represents purity. It can be perceived as hygienic and sterile which is why it's used in hospitals and clinics worldwide.

GREY: A neutral colour. Grey can have a dampening effect on other colours and can indicate a lack of confidence. However, charcoal grey may be a great alternative for suiting if black is too harsh for you.

Your clothes can also have an effect when you need to modify others' perception of you to get the best result.

EXERCISE: YOUR PERSONALITY

First of all I'd like you to think about your own personality. Where would you sit on a scale of 1 – 10 with shy at 1 and authoritative at 10? Are there certain circumstances when it would be beneficial to move up or down the scale to appear more or less domineering?

The way you put your clothes together can help you to achieve this.

One of my clients is a teacher. She works in a school where discipline is often difficult to achieve. She is expected to get great results at GCE and, on the whole, she achieves this with hard work and dedication. She had recently begun to notice, however, that her pupils were taking little notice of what she was saying or doing. Her control of the class was diminishing and it was causing her distress.

We looked at her chosen style of dress. She was wearing a full length 'boho' skirt with lots of layers, teamed with a logo' T-shirt, gold belt and flip-flop type sandals. She looked extremely trendy and the look suited both her figure and her personality.

However, by dressing in this way, she looked more like one of her pupils rather than their teacher.

We needed to create a look that was still modern and up to date but also said, "listen to me – I'm in charge." I suggested that she wore a pair of cropped (or normal length) trousers with a matching waistcoat and a victoriana blouse in a contrasting colour. We teamed this with a pair of boots and we pinned back her hair. The result? She still felt trendy but her class instantly knew that she was in charge. No more authority problems for her.

Whether or not you work for a living, it is crucial to your well-being that you have great relationships with other people. Apparently, 85% of our problems are caused by people that we don't see eye to eye with and the way you dress can once again come to your assistance. So here are some tips that will help you dress appropriately for an interaction with someone else:

1. Authority is gained by wearing clothes with maximum contrast: black and white, dark brown and cream, navy and palest blue.

2. A softer image is gained by dressing in tones and shades of a single colour: brown or green trousers with slightly lighter shade for the upper body.

3. Plain, bold colour is authoritative.

4. Introduce pattern or design for a softer look.

5.   A jacket that compliments, but doesn't exactly match, your trousers or skirt will appear less authoritative.

6.   Fabrics that are stiff and starchy will appear more authoritative than those that have more fluidity and drape. The same applies to garments with lots of fitted tailoring (authority) and less structure (approachable). A cardigan/twinset worn with trousers or a skirt will show less authority than a suit.

7.   Red and/or black can look powerful. Pastels will appear less so.

8.   Hairstyles that are severe will give an impression of power. The same applies to your spectacles. Black rimmed glasses are more authoritative than rimless ones.

Face Facts

"There are no ugly women. Every woman is a Venus in her own way."

Brigitte Bardot - Actress

Your face is probably the most important part of your body. It's often the first thing we notice about someone, whether in a business meeting or across a crowded room.

If you're like me then you'll probably only notice the "bad" bits. Your concentration will be on whether you have more wrinkles, bags under your eyes or spots.

Understanding the shape of your face and your features will help you to flatter what nature gave you. This in turn will enhance your natural beauty and good looks. You'll be able to choose hairstyles, specs and jewellery that really do you justice and keep you looking up to date.

Whatever your face shape, the biggest hint I can give you to looking beautiful is simple. Just SMILE.

Step 1:

Using a mirror, look at your facial features.

- Is your nose long and straight or is it small, short or full?

- Do your eyebrows sit straight or are they arched?

- Are your eyes small and/or almond shaped or are they large and round?

- Do you have visible cheekbones and planes within your face or are your cheeks soft and rounded?

- Are your lips thin and straight or plump and large?

- Is your chin square and/or angular or is it soft and/or rounded?

Keep your mirror handy as you'll need this later.

If you answered mostly yes to the first answer in each of the questions then you have angular features. If you answered mostly yes to the second answers then your features are contoured.

You may remember we touched on these terms when looking at body shapes. Don't worry if your features are different to your body shape. It is possible to have a body that is one shape and a face that is another.

If you have long hair then tie it back so that the outline of your face is visible. Starting at the top of your head, use both hands to trace the outline with your fingertips so you can really see its shape. Is it wide or long? Do you have a pronounced jawline?

On the whole, people with angular features will have a square or rectangular face. Contoured features normally reside in an oval or round face.

It's time to go back to the art of illusion again.

If your face is very narrow then it helps to make it appear wider. Conversely, if it's wide then we need to lengthen it.

Long Faces

Best suit hairstyles that provide some width. A high pony tail or lots of hair on top of the head will only add to the illusion of length, as will very long straight hair. Create balance by having more hair at the sides of your face or curling the hair out and way from the face. Use blow drying to add volume at the sides. If your jaw is pointed then hair will look great if wide at this point as it will detract attention away.

Spectacles and sunglasses should fit outside the contours of the face. This provides a horizontal line that shortens and widens.

If you have a long nose then choose plastic rather than metal frames. The thicker, dark bridge will shorten it.

Avoid long dangly earrings as these will also drag the eye downwards. Look for earrings that are wide and sit at ear level.

Wide faces:

Need to look longer so hairstyles with height on the top or length at the bottom will help. Square jaws can be complemented by longer styles and a side fringe. A jaw length bob and a straight fringe can appear a little like curtains in a window frame.

Spectacles should sit inside the contours of the face. A high bridge in metal will lengthen the nose if required.

Earrings that are long and dangly, or hoops that appear long when viewed from the front will add required length to the face.

On the whole, general style principles apply just as they did to your body shape. If you have an angular face then think stiff fabrics around the neck, geometric shaped glasses and sharp haircuts.

Contoured faces need more softness and look good with wavier hair, slightly curved frames and softer fabrics round the neck.

GONE TO YOUR HEAD!

Guidelines for hairstyles and spectacles (including sunglasses)

Oval:

Probably the most versatile of all the face shapes, with evenly proportioned features and width at cheek bone level. Naomi Campbell has this face shape.

- You can carry off almost any style – lucky you – but hair that is too short may make the face appear longer.

- You can also wear most jewellery and spectacles well.

Round:

This face shape is similar in height and width with full cheeks and a rounded jawline. Arabella Weir has this face shape.

- You will need to make your face look longer so you suit hairstyles with height or length. A layered cut using gel, a high pony tail/topknot or longer hair left loose all work well.

- Spectacles should sit inside the outline of the face to narrow. A thin bridge will lengthen the nose. Avoid round styles though as you will look like an owl!

- Earrings should be worn long to add length to the face.

Heart:
With this face shape, the forehead and cheekbones are wide while the jaw and chin are narrow. Sophie Dahl has this face shape.

- You need to balance the face by adding width to the lower half.

- Bobs worn between chin and shoulder length, with a side parting or side fringe look great. Avoid harsh short cuts or height on the top of the head. Keep wispy bits at the base of the neck to balance.

- The best spectacles have frames which accentuate the bottom. Half glasses, which have a coloured rim at the bottom and clear glass at the top look fantastic on a heart shaped face.

- Earrings should have some additional width.

Pear:

With this face shape, the widest point is at ear level while the jaw is quite defined and the forehead narrow. Minnie Driver and Jennifer Aniston have this face shape.

- You need to make the forehead wider.

- Hair should be kept close at the sides, have some height and weight on top (to balance the jawline) and be kept off the forehead.

- Frames should be heavier on the top than the bottom and be slightly rounded.

- Earrings should be long but not too wide.

Square:

This face shape is identified by straight sides, a wide forehead and very square jawline. Cherie Blair has this face shape.

- You need to narrow and soften your face.

- Avoid a fringe with chin length bob because it can look like curtains!

- Asymmetrical fringes look softer. Hair should be shoulder length or have height on the top of the head. Avoid width at the sides.

- Frames should be narrower than the face. High sides and bridge will add length.

- Earrings should be long and not wide

Rectangle:
This face shape is relatively long with straight sides and a wide forehead. It can have sharp jaw or a softer one. Nicole Kidman has this face shape.

- You need to balance the length by creating width.

- Hair should be full to provide width. Alternatively, a fringe (full or partial) will reduce length.

- Spectacles should be wider than the outline of the face. This creates a horizontal line which widens and shortens.

- Earrings should be wide not long.

Diamond:
With this face shape the cheeks are the widest point and the forehead and chin are narrower. Most often seen in Asian women.

- You need to widen both forehead and chin.

- Hair should create fullness at the back. A side parting or side fringe will help disguise a narrow forehead.

- Specs should be narrower than the outline of the face.

- Earrings should be wide.

Triangle:
This face shape will taper to a narrow chin making the forehead look wide. Victoria Beckham has this face shape.

- You need to create width around chin area.

- Hair should add visual width at the back of the head.

- Spectacles should be narrower than the outline of the face. If possible, they should be wider on the bottom than the top.

- Earrings should add width and long styles should be avoided.

As I have a very long face, I use my oversize spectacles to shorten. It really does work, and they also hide the bags under my eyes! Talking of which...

THE EYES HAVE IT

If you are a spectacle wearer then you need to be aware that your whole look can rest on how well your glasses suit you. Glasses can add impact (Jenny Éclair) or be almost invisible if they are frameless.

Think about what you want your glasses to say about you and choose accordingly.

Generally speaking, if you have cool skin you will suit silver, black, blue, purple or burgundy frames. If you're a warm skinned person then you'll look better in gold, tortoiseshell, brown or red.

Metal frames with a high bridge will elongate the nose. Plastic frames with a solid bridge will make the nose look shorter.

The shape of your specs depends on your face shape.

An angular face will suit geometric frames. A rounder face will need frames that have a slight curve. Owl type glasses are a definite no-no for everyone! This also applies to sunglasses.

Lenses that change colour according to the light used to scream 'old fashioned', but there are some really subtle ones on the market now. If your eyes are sensitive to light then take a look – they may be just what you need.

If you haven't changed your specs for a couple of years then you may be in danger of looking dated or frumpy. There are so many styles to choose from now and many opticians offer a 2nd pair free. There is really no excuse not to try on some new styles and update your look.

Hair Raising

"I think the most important thing a woman can have – next to talent of course – is her hairdresser."

Joan Crawford, Actress

Your hair is your shining glory. I think it's fair to say that if we have a bad hair day, our whole life is put on hold. We know logically that it will grow again but it seems that it might take a lifetime to do so!

How long is it since you had a good look at your hair? Is the style current? Does it suit you or have you not changed it for a number of years? Do you have it coloured or highlighted? Is it manageable? Does it suit your lifestyle?

A good hairdresser will ask all of these questions and more. To ensure that the hair is in proportion to your height, a professional hairstylist should ask you to stand up before making any decisions about the style and cut.

It's vital that your hair suits your lifestyle. You don't want a complicated creation if you have small children to look after or you are a 'wash and go' type of woman. So make sure your hairdresser understands this

The shape of your face can also help you decide which way to wear your hair (see Face Facts). A rounder, contoured face needs a softer style. If you have cheekbones and are more angled, you can sport a sharper look. A long, thin face can benefit from hair with width. A short, wide face needs height on top or a longer length to create slimness and length.

Look also at the texture of your hair. If it's going grey and is very dry, it might benefit from a shorter cut. We all aspire to lustrous, long locks but if we haven't got them, there are other ways to make your hairstyle work for you. Long hair can be ageing.

If you are losing your hair due to the menopause or illness, the most important thing to do is make sure that you have a really good cut. Long hair tends to drag and will pull on the scalp making the hair loss appear worse. A shortish style, perhaps with some length on the top of the head if required, will minimise the exposure. Keep the application of hair products to a minimum. Too much wax will add weight to the hair shaft and make the problem worse. Buy the very best product you can afford to thicken the hair and then use sparingly. Colour can also help. A tint or semi permanent colour can add gloss and shine so the hair appears fuller.

Anyone can look more stylish and trendy by the introduction of a few colour highlights, some wax to gift lift or a choppy cut to give a funky look. It doesn't have to take oodles of time. – just a few minutes daily effort can take years off you. I'm terrible with hair so I have worn it short for years. No curling tongues or straightening irons have ever graced my dressing table. I blast it with a hairdryer and apply some wax. Stylish and funky in 5 minutes flat.

You can make the most of your hair by pampering yourself. There are products on the market that act like a masque, providing intensive moisture to make the hair shaft look sleek and shiny. Buy shampoos and conditioners that suit your hair type and try to wash your hair on a daily basis. Massaging your scalp can bring much needed blood to the surface of the scalp. Not only is this therapeutic but it will enhance the condition of your hair.

If you are suffering from a time warp where your hair is concerned, do yourself a favour and book a free consultation now. Ask for recommendations from friends or colleagues who have hair that always looks good. You don't have to go to an expensive salon.

Some of the best hairdressers I've come across are mobile, and consequently, very affordable.

The relationship with your hairdresser is precious. Trust is vital. If you speak to one that doesn't quite resonate with you, don't feel afraid to visit someone else. You won't regret it.

Kiss & Make Up

"The best thing is to look natural, but it takes make-up to look natural."

Calvin Klein - Couturier

I'm pretty sure that our postman thinks that my husband has two different women living at our house.

Normally, he arrives very early with our mail, about 6.30am, and I am the one who goes to collect it from him. The sight must be quite frightening actually – hair standing on end like I've just electrocuted myself, eye bags like a Bassett Hound and the wrinkles of a Staffordshire Bull Terrier – no disrespect to any dogs out there!

I remember vividly the day he came late with a parcel to be signed for. By this time I was dressed and fully made up. When I opened the door, he stepped back in amazement. I could hear him thinking – this cannot be the woman who usually comes to the door.

I could have got very upset about this. I am well aware of how old my skin is looking. Too many years of sunbathing with olive oil, poor eating habits, alcohol and stress have all shown up in my face.

I recently visited a face reader. She told me that the horizontal lines on my forehead were signs of mental agility and curiosity for life. My eyes, despite the bags, showed natural enthusiasm, openness, tolerance and that I was easy to get along with. I liked what she said.

Would I still be the same if I'd been botoxed I wonder? This is my face and it tells my story. I'm not sure that I would be happy with one that didn't say anything about the real me.

Well dear reader, if I can turn myself around, so can you. We can all scrub up well if we know what we are doing.

I'm not advocating that you should wear make up all the time though. A beautician friend of mine never wears makeup while she's working. She has niched herself as a 'holistic' beautician and she is very successful.

If you too have great skin and know you look attractive au-naturel, just use this chapter for those special occasions. You may need to know, however, that research has shown that women who ware carefully applied make up for work do tend to earn up to 20% more than their bare faced colleagues.

PAINT A PICTURE

It's unfortunate, but as we get older, our skin loses colour, it sags and it wrinkles. That's a fact. It doesn't mean that the world has ended though.

These days, cosmetic houses are working hard to produce creams and cosmetics to suit a more mature complexion. Light diffusing foundations, moisturising lipsticks and lip glosses can all help create the illusion of young, healthy skin.

As a rule of thumb, the following basic principles will enable you to apply your makeup in a way that enhances your complexion.

Foundation:

Foundation is probably the hardest item to buy correctly. It is the base for all your makeup and is used to even out your skin tone NOT to add colour to it. Buy only after you have seen it on your skin in broad daylight.

A beautician friend of mine always says that you would never buy a shoe by trying it on your hand! It's the same with foundation. It should be placed around jaw level, not on your hand, as the skin is totally different in colour and texture. Wait for a few minutes to let it absorb. There should be no discernible difference.

Apply your foundation all over the skin including the eye area. This will enable any eye shadow to stay in place for longer. Make sure it is well blended into the skin, especially around the jaw and hairline. If you want a more natural look then you can blend it with moisturiser, or use a damp sponge to give less coverage.

I find that foundation covers more naturally if you start from the centre of the face and blend outwards. This way you have less left on the sponge or your fingertips when you reach your hairline. There is nothing worse than seeing too much depth of colour in the hair or at jaw level.

These days you can buy light diffusing foundations that are supposed to make us look younger. They are light in texture but still give a good coverage. Heavier foundations can sit in the wrinkles of the skin so beware.

Concealer:

Used to hide blemishes and dark under eye circles, it can be a godsend if applied correctly. I always apply after my foundation, because the foundation may have done the job well enough.

For under eye circles, use a light creamy formulation so it won't drag the delicate skin under the eye. Dap it on using your ring finger, as it has less power than your index finger and we don't want you poking your eye out!

A concealer with yellow undertones will camouflage blue veins under the skin. Otherwise opt for one with light diffusing properties and dab gently on affected areas.

If you have high colour, a green cream will disguise the redness. This will also work on pimples that are red and angry looking. Don't choose one that is too greasy though or it will make the problem worse.

Darker spots or moles need a heavier consistency. A stick or pencil is your best choice.

Powder:

Buy a fine, translucent powder as a setting agent. Dab over your face with the powder puff. Remove excess by using a large brush with downward strokes. If you have wrinkles then buy the finest texture you can find – otherwise it will show up in the lines on your face. If you want a tanned effect then use a bronzer with a large brush and sweep over the face.

Blusher:

You can find both cream and powder blushers on the market. I tend to stick with a fine powder as the cream seems to make me look a bit like Aunt Sally from Worzel Gummidge.

To apply blusher – smile. Using a brush, start from the apple of your cheek and blend upwards and backwards towards the hair line. To ensure you're not heavy handed hold the brush loosely between thumb and 1st and 2nd fingers and not as if you were holding a pencil and shake any excess onto a tissue before application. For a special evening look lightly brush the forehead, nose and chin with blusher to highlight the T zone.

Eyebrows:

Eyebrows act as a frame for your face. Take a pencil and hold it by the side of your nose, and by the inner corner of your eye. Where the tip ends is where your eyebrow should start. Take the pencil tip towards the outer corner of your eye and this indicates where your brow should end. Take a grey or brown pencil (or use eyeshadow and a brush) and use feather like strokes to fill in any gaps. If you are using powder, go against the direction of hair growth for best results.

Make sure you keep your eyebrows in good shape, either by plucking, waxing or threading. Really unruly eyebrow hairs can be professionally removed by electrolysis. Always remove stray hairs from the bottom and never the top of the brow. Pull skin taughtly between your fingers and tweeze out in the direction of the hair growth. It's often a good idea to colour in the perfect eyebrow first. This will provide a template so stray hairs can be easily spotted. Clear mascara can help keep unruly hairs in place.

Eyes:

Eyeshadow looks better if it's not too pearly or iridescent, as these qualities can highlight any wrinkling. Bright greens and blues should be left to the young. Try neutral colours with a brighter eye pencil to add interest. Eye pencils should be applied with light, feathery strokes to define the area underneath the eye and in the outer corners.

Finish the look with a coat of mascara. Again, unless you're very dark, avoid black and opt for grey or black/brown. Many cosmetic houses now do stunning shades of turquoise and purple if you want a different and dramatic look.

To use mascara to its best advantage, look down and lightly brush the top side of your upper lashes first. This will provide length. Then looking straight at the mirror, brush the underside upwards.

If you wear mascara on your lower lashes then use a zigzag motion with the wand first. Then you can brush downwards to get length and volume if required.

If your eyelashes are sparse then use an eyelash conditioner first. This will provide moisture and add thickness. If they are very straight then use an eyelash curler to open up the eye area before applying your mascara.

If you have eyes set wide apart, your eye pencil should run 2/3 of the lower lid, working from the outer corner. If they are narrow set, use only 1/3 and blend well. This will make the eyes appear to be spaced wider apart.

If you have little or no eyelids, dispense with eyeliner. It will make the eyelids look heavy and you will look tired. Use a lighter colour instead to open them up.

A prominent brow bone should not be highlighted with a light colour as it will make it stand out even more. Instead use a colour that almost matches your skin tone so it recedes.

Lips:

Our lip lines often get blurred as we age – especially if we smoke. There are special products on the market to counteract this and they are well worth investing in. Lips can often get thinner too. If so, don't choose a lip colour that is too dark as it will make them look even smaller.

To outline the lip area, choose a lip pencil that is close to your own lip colour, rather than one that matches your lipstick. This will provide a better outline and can make the lips look larger if required. It will also prevent feathering, where the lipstick gets drawn into the tiny lines around the mouth. Don't try to draw the lip outline in one go, as it will often look clownish. Firstly, draw in your cupid's bow. Then take the pencil and draw in the equivalent distance on your bottom lip. You can then connect the dots moving from the centre to the corner of the mouth. Use a lip brush to apply your lipstick or gloss. To keep lipstick on your lips, blot with a tissue and then re-apply.

Remember to choose cosmetics that suit your complexion and your colouring (see Face Facts). Opt for rose tones if cool and coral if warm. If you are dark then you can wear deeper shades than if you are fair. If you are bright then you can wear brighter lipstick. If you are muted it's best to stick to softer shades.

Cleansing:

I have no wish to teach grandmothers to suck eggs so to speak, so forgive me if your cleansing routine has been maintained for years. It becomes even more important as we get older and the oestrogen levels change, that you don't skimp on looking after your skin.

Cleanse, tone and moisturise with products suitable for your skin type at least once a day. This will help you to retain the dewiness and freshness of younger skin. One with SPF15 minimum will prevent further damage from the sun. Lastly, ALWAYS take off your makeup before going to bed. Who wants to wake up to dirty pillowcases anyway?

Talking of pillowcases, I have been reliably informed that silk ones prevent the face wrinkling from sleep and also keep your hairstyle intact. You'll have to test that one out for yourself!

If you so desire, you can use a face mask after exfoliating on a weekly basis. Be careful if your skin is delicate or very dry that the exfoliating scrub is not too harsh for your skin.

I often apply vitamin E oil as I feel that it sinks into my skin and nourishes it really well. If you do it prior to going to sleep you will wake up with gorgeously soft skin.

Day creams tend to be lighter than night creams, as all the repair work is done while we are in bed. Be careful of putting too much around the eyes as it can make them puffy. Specialist eye creams should be used for this purpose, dabbed on the top of the cheek bone gently using the ring finger so the skin doesn't get dragged and damaged.

With fluctuating oestrogen levels, you may find that your skin will become much drier or much oilier. If this is the case, you will need to change your skin creams accordingly.

DARE TO BARE

Don't forget the rest of your body too. A weekly exfoliate plus moisturising daily can be of great help to the skin covering the rest of you. If that's too much trouble then run yourself a bath and soak in some luxurious oils with a glass of champagne at your side. Alternatively, treat yourself to a massage. You know you're worth it!

Cellulite:

Much has been made of cellulite – those bumpy lumps under the skin – usually around the bottom and the back of the thighs. Some doctors swear it doesn't exist but I know many people who believe differently.

If you do have these orange peel type lumps then you can try body brushing. Use a bristle body brush in circular motions, moving towards the heart. Do this before showering and hopefully, you may notice a difference. There are specialist creams on the market that you could try too. Drinking plenty of water and regular exercise may also help alleviate the problem.

Stretch Marks:

Applying a vitamin E oil or cream can help reduce stretch marks. Don't expect miracles overnight. Your skin will feel really soft though.

NAIL BITING

Ragged or unkempt nails can really let you down. Following the trend set in the USA, many nail bars have been set up around the country. So there is no longer any excuse for having dodgy digits.

Home Manicure:

- Soak your nails for 5 minutes then remove existing polish with cotton wool and nail polish remover.

- Clip nails straight across. Pointed nails are weaker.

- File nails, working from outside in. They should be square with slightly rounded edges.

- Apply cuticle remover and soften hands in water for 3 minutes.

- Wrap cotton wool around an orangewood/manicure stick and GENTLY push back cuticles. Wash your hands.

- Apply base coat before applying nail colour and a final top coat.

Home Pedicure:

Feet are something we really take for granted. Think how you would manage if something happened to them and you couldn't walk. It's time to give them some recognition and a well-earned pampering session. I couldn't live without my foot spa and my feet say "thank you" too.

- Soak nails for 5 minutes. Take off existing polish with cotton wool and nail polish remover.

- Clip nails straight across and file if necessary towards the centre with single strokes.

- Buff the surface of the nail to remove ridges.

- Apply cuticle remover and soak feet for about 3 minutes – add lemon juice if nails are stained.

- Gently push back cuticles using an orangewood/manicure stick wrapped with cotton wool.

- Use an exfoliator to remove dry skin on backs of heels or to soften any callouses.

- Dry feet thoroughly and apply a rich foot cream.

- Separate toes with tissue and apply a base coat. When dry, apply colour and a top coat.

GIRL POWER

If you still need convincing that applying make up can give you a real boost then the following might help change your mind.

I work as a volunteer for a charity called Look Good Feel Better (www.lgfb.co.uk). They organise a number of workshops in major hospitals throughout the UK for ladies who have undergone treatment for cancer.

During these workshops, my colleagues and I teach the ladies how to apply makeup step by step. The transformation is amazing. They not only look fantastic but also their excitement and enthusiasm levels have gone through the roof.

The buzz in the atmosphere is tremendous. They definitely leave the room with a completely different attitude to when they first came in. If you are a makeup virgin then have a go and see what the power of makeup can do for you.

Sue Donnelly

Who Are You?

"Why not be oneself? That is the whole secret of a successful appearance. If one is a greyhound, why try to look like a Pekinese?"

Edith Sitwell, Poet

FINDING THE REAL YOU

Now we get down to the real nitty gritty. So far you've established your overall body and face shape, the colours that best suit you and how to disguise any figure challenges. Well done for getting this far.

This chapter is all about dressing yourself in an authentic way. It's no good following the rules, if you don't feel comfortable with the overall result. Clothes should be an extension of your personality and not a suit of armour or a mask. Don't think designer labels are the answer either; it's the congruency between you and your clothing that gives you power and not the label on show.

I have a slim, angular body and the expertise to make my legs appear much longer than they are. In theory, I would look good wearing a short leather mini skirt, high heels and fishnet stockings.

However, this style of dress does not fit in with my overall values. The result – I would look and feel uncomfortable, lose my confidence and probably bolt for the nearest hiding place. This is even more alarming when you understand that 'talking' to people is one of my pleasures in life and I'm very well practiced!

A client of mine works in an office environment where suits are the norm for both men and women. She is a larger than life, bubbly person and the idea of her in a buttoned up suit just does not sit well.

Between us, we've managed to create a look that fits in with her corporate lifestyle but also expresses her own unique personality. Instead of using pin-stripes and severe tailoring in her clothing, she has selected a less structured style of suit. She wears this with brightly coloured blouses with frilly collars in drapey fabrics. She looks professional, but also liberated at the same time. Her hair is left loose or pinned back, with tendrils to soften her face. She looks fantastic and radiates confidence.

Guess what, she also is highly successful. Because she looks and feels confident, she attracts colleagues and clients who want to work with her. All good news for the bottom line.

Step 1:

Think about the words you would use to describe yourself. Make a list, group them and then narrow it down to 2 or 3 key adjectives. These will be your values. Take your time over this as it's the key to finding the real you.

My 3 Key Words are:

1..

2..

3..

Step 2:

Look at your style of dress. Does it fully express the words you've just used about yourself? If not then why not?

For instance, if one of your key descriptors is 'enthusiastic', it will come across more successfully with a wardrobe full of colour rather than all black clothing. If it's 'honest' then perhaps some earthier tones may be useful.

My current style of dress is:

....

....

....

....

Step 3:

Ask someone you trust to describe you. Are the adjectives they use the same as yours? If not then ask them why they see you differently. Does your style have anything to do with it? Are your clothes giving out the wrong impression?

My friend's descriptors of me are:

1...

2...

3...

YOUR STYLE PREFERENCES

We are all unique – so trying to copy a style just because it suits someone else is nigh on impossible. The following will help you understand the way you prefer to dress. It will also help you realise that your shopping habits and wardrobe management may be totally different from those around you.

Think about the following:

a. Do you covet the latest trends and constantly change your look?

b. Do you prefer quality tailoring that allows easy coordination of your clothes?

c. Do you love pretty, feminine clothes and prefer skirts to trousers?

d. Are you a "wash 'n' go" type of person who opts for a more natural, relaxed look?

e. Do you create a statement by using the unusual, such as a great piece of jewellery, a funky hairstyle or clothes in strong colour combinations?

Choose the description above that is most like you as it will be a key indicator of how your personality is reflected through your attire.

If you are most like answer **a**, then you are a **creative** dresser. The best type of shopping for you is rummaging through charity shops and vintage stores to find eclectic items which you can throw together. Chain stores hold no appeal as they are too 'mass market'. You crave individuality and artistry.

If you resonated with answer **b**, then you are a **classic** dresser. You love garments that stand the test of time and always look smart due to their tailoring. Rarely are textures or colours mixed as you prefer a coordinated approach to dressing. You will hardly ever (if at all) be spotted wearing jeans or cords. Fashion trends do not interest you at all.

If you selected **c** as your answer, then you are a feminine dresser and masculine attire does not interest you. You are a **romantic** dresser. Pretty colours, florals, patterns and floaty fabrics are the essence of your wardrobe. Your clothes may not be too structured but you will pay attention to the detail.

If you picked **d** as the answer most like you, then you are a **casual** dresser. You may have leanings towards sporty clothes such as trainers and T-shirts, rather than high heels and blouses, or just prefer natural fabrics with little or no structure. Relaxed and comfortable are your key words. You will wear minimal jewellery and little or no makeup, with hair tied back or flowing loose around your face.

The answer **e** reflects a **dramatic** dresser. You create attention by using unique and individual accessories or by bold use of colour. You may be high-maintenance and you may also have lots of clothes that have only been worn once; you couldn't possibly wear it again – someone may have seen it before! Clothes make a statement about you and, even if you're not aware of it, you will be noticed.

Make the most of your style by choosing garments and accessories that fit in with your natural personality.

- **Creative** dressers can choose belts, scarves that don't coordinate, vintage pieces, unusual brooches or corsages, crocheted shrugs, feather boas or anything that looks slightly eccentric to show off their look to the maximum. Mixing textures such as wool and chiffon can also work as long as it doesn't add unwanted bulk. Be careful not to make excessive purchases that mean items never get worn. If you want to follow the trends then make sure you adapt them to your age and body line.

- **Classic** dressers can mix and match existing garments with any new purchases. Try to vary your look by bringing in some colour. Simplicity and understatement are key to your look so beware of wearing too many pieces of jewellery at once. Although you may prefer the real thing, try good quality costume jewellery if you want to add some variety. To modernise, change your hosiery to flesh coloured fishnets or a softly patterned dark opaque. Handbags and shoes should no longer match exactly so keep the colours the same but change fabric types. Make sure that your garments are classic and not dated, if you want to look youthful.

- **Romantic** dressers can look great in garments that have some appliqué, beading or diamante. Soft layers, floaty fabrics and frills in chiffon or lace are your style. Select luxurious fabrics such as cashmere, satin and silk, for both outer wear and underwear. Soft, pretty cardigans or shrugs may look better than a jacket. Floral prints and abstracts can work well too but remember your scale and don't overdo it. Woven or decorative handbags look better than stiff leather. Don't forget your heels – as if you would!

- **Natural** dressers look best in natural fabrics and neutral colours. For you, linen, wool, suede and leather in loose fitting styles will make the best jackets. Choose comfortable shoes but try to make them modern – ballet pumps, for instance, can look great with jeans or a skirt. Gilets, boot cut trousers and wrap cardigans are easy to wear and can look natural and stylish at the same time. If you must have elasticated waists then make sure they don't bulk and give you bumps where you don't want them. Remember though, that being relaxed is not the same as not making an effort. A pair of pearl earrings, some mascara and lip gloss can provide extra glamour when required.

- **Dramatic** dressers need to look for key pieces that add impact. Wear unusual buckles on your belt, eye catching spectacles, a huge ring, a unique bag or killer shoes. Only one or two though – don't overdo it or you'll look like a Christmas tree! Alternatively, add a streak of colour to your hair, wear coloured mascara and paint your lips in bright or dark red or pink. Bold colours suit your style and your attitude.

So using this information, together with your 3 key descriptors, please answer the following:

Step 4:

What can you do to dress in a more authentic manner? Could you introduce something new to update your look or throw out garments that are alien to your nature?

....

....

....

....

HOME IS WHERE THE HEART IS

If you're still unclear about what your style consists of then take a look at your home. A person's interior décor can often represent the real them.

My home tends to be quite colourful but minimalistic. There is no wallpaper, just painted walls. No chintz or frills or flounces. Every room has one eye catching feature – an unusual painting or an elegant chair. I tend to spend money on the basics, such as a leather suite, and they will be in neutral tones. The accessories will provide any colour. This has the added advantage of making it easy to change the look of the room without spending too much money.

The essence of my home reflects the essential style elements of my dress sense. I never wear much jewellery, just a statement piece that will be very different. My clothes are colourful but never frilly or flouncy. My look is quite understated but bold, just like my house.

One of my clients has a beautiful, modern and airy home. All surfaces and walls are white. The only colour comes from some fabulous artwork that she has painted herself. She had contacted me because she had lost sight of her identity and had no concept of what would suit her now that she was older. Her clothes – black, black and more black were often shapeless with no uniqueness or charisma. Once she had realised that her own style preferences existed, albeit within her home, she could transfer the guidelines into her wardrobe. She now dresses in light neutrals, using bright jewellery and lipstick as her colour accents. She sparkles and looks radiant.

So, have a fresh look at your own home. What does it say about you? If you are not living in a home that suits your personal taste at this present time then imagine one that would and carry out the exercise using this as your template.

GETTING THE BALANCE RIGHT

As human beings, we are multi-dimensional and so is our day to day existence. The various roles we play of mother, breadwinner, aunt, grandma, friend, partner and so on require different types of clothes. Many occasions also call for completely different attire. A balanced wardrobe requires clothes that can serve us for all aspects of our life.

To find out if your wardrobe is working for you, do the following exercise.

Take a piece of paper and draw two circles.

Using the circle as a pi chart, divide it into sections proportionate to the different areas of your life (excluding sleeping time). For instance, 40% may be work, 25% gym, 15% socialising, 10% gardening, 10% pottering about the house and so on.

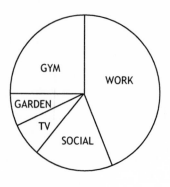

In the second circle, do the same thing with the clothes you own. For example, 25% of your clothes are suits, 10% are jeans, 30% sweaters and so on.

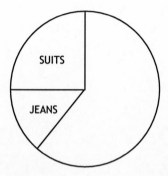

Now compare the results. Do they marry up or has one area totally dominated your wardrobe? Ask yourself why that might be. What are you hanging onto? What are you trying to avoid? If it does match up then well done – you've got it just right.

Using all the information you learned about yourself (your personality, your style preferences and your work/life wardrobe requirements), complete the next step.

Step 5:

Are your clothes appropriate for your personality, your style preferences and your lifestyle? Do your clothes reflect the image that you want to project – at work and in your social life? Have you got the balance right between work and play? What changes do you need to make?

....

....

....

....

As the Greek Philosopher, Epicetus once said: "Know first who you are and then adorn yourself accordingly."

Suits You

"By itself reality per se isn't worth a damn. It's perception that promotes reality to meaning."

Joseph Brodsky - Academic

Each one of us has an image whether we actively cultivate one or not. The way you present yourself to the rest of the world is the way you will be viewed. Whether that view is valid or not is up to you.

All of us make initial judgements about people in seconds - their background, how much they earn, how educated they are and so on. Humans are programmed to believe first what we see rather than what we hear, so our reference in this process centres round the visual.

What we actually say only accounts for very little (7%) of what people think about us. Non-verbal signals, body language, eye contact, confidence, height, weight, colouring, clothing, hairstyles and accessories account for a massive 93%, of which 55% concentrates on our visual appearance alone.

Your image, therefore, is crucial in terms of your career progress, an interview, a first date or any event that's important to you.

In the corporate world there is a phenomenon known as "The Spiral of Success". When you look good, you feel good and your self-esteem increases. As a result, this will enable you to project yourself with more conviction and confidence. Others will be more drawn to you, so you are likely to gain more positive responses from work associates, family, friends and even strangers. From a business stance you are more likely to gain trust and respect. The result – a positive impact on your relationships and, ultimately, your bottom line.

As 90% of our bodies are covered by clothes – it would seem logical to dress them in the best way possible. This book should be helping you to do just that. It will give you the chance to look at the basics in an unthreatening way. It will tell you things your best friend might not. It will help you to understand what really suits you, what to wear and when to wear it. If you know you look good then your image is one less thing to worry about meaning you can focus on the things that really matter to you.

Remember: just because you looked great in something years ago it does not mean that it is still appropriate today. A dated look may also be interpreted as 'behind the times' in the workplace too.

Remaining authentic and true to yourself is fundamental to your success. Your 'self' is what you are all about. Understanding how to acquire an image that conveys your true essence to the people around you is the critical factor.

However, there are other factors to take into consideration when dressing in a business environment:

APPROPRIATENESS

Your attire must be appropriate; not only for the occasion and your audience but also your objectives, your industry and the situation itself. You would not expect to find a tattooed waitress serving in an upmarket restaurant for example.

One of my clients is a Personal Life Coach. She had only just started in her new profession after leaving the banking world and she couldn't understand why her client list was dwindling. On looking at her attire – it suddenly became obvious. She was wearing the same outfit she would have worn to the bank. The pin striped look was not appropriate for her new clientele, who needed a much softer image for them to feel comfortable.

Admittedly, there are some professions where you must stick to the rules. In the legal profession, for instance, a court appearance will mean a black suit and white shirt. Whether or not it suits your personal colouring is irrelevant.

YOUR 'BRAND'

In the chapter entitled, 'Who Are You?', there is an exercise to discover your values and how you utilise them to best effect in your dress. Why is it important? Well, if there are two equally qualified and experienced people applying for the same job or contract then their 'brand' is what will tell them apart. For instance, imagine two women applying for the same role within a company and their CV's are practically identical. If one wears well applied makeup and the other doesn't, it's highly likely that the make up wearer will get the job. Why? Because it is perceived that she has made the extra effort. In fact, on the subject of makeup, a woman wearing makeup can expect to earn up to 20% more than her bare faced sisters.

Even in promotional terms, image counts for 30% of getting the new position. Only 10% is geared around your ability to do the job and 60% is centred on networking and promoting yourself. The latter cannot be done without a good personal image.

PERSONAL ATTIRE

Your outfit should suit your body shape, your colouring, your scale and your personality. For more information on these topics, please look at the relevant chapters.

DO YOUR RESEARCH

If you are looking for funding, applying for a new job, presenting to a group and so on then it's essential that you do your research beforehand. The banking profession is synonymous with pin-striped suiting; the advertising industry is not. Check what you are expected to wear beforehand.

A client once told me of her husband's misfortune at being turned down for a loan. He works in advertising and had gone to the bank in his normal 'uniform' of black shirt and black jeans. While it is perfectly reasonable to wear this type of outfit in the advertising world – the bank didn't quite see it in the same light. Her husband had not given enough thought to *who* he was meeting, the environment in which they worked and the occasion. He was going to them for money and he needed to dress according to their expectations and not his own.

FRAGRANCE

I'm not talking about personal hygiene because I'm assuming that will be in order. I'm talking about perfume. I've actually stopped wearing it for meetings now. Smell can be strongly associated with memories and the emotions they evoke. Even if your scent isn't overpowering, you don't want to remind someone of somebody else they didn't get on with! So it's best to leave it off if you haven't met before.

GROOMING

It goes without saying that you should always be well groomed for an important event. This does not mean wearing nail varnish at all times but it does mean having well kept nails. Hair should be clean and tidy and in a style that suits both you and the situation. A soft look will not work well if you want to come across as smart and decisive. The chapter 'It's not All Black and White' will help you to choose powerful colours if required.

ETIQUETTE

Learn how to shake hands well if you haven't already. A perfect handshake should meet web to web and be firm. Try it out on your friends to check that you are not too limp-wristed or crushing bones.

Be sure not to get too close. People feel intimidated if you invade their personal space. 'Personal space' is usually defined as 18 inches around the body.

Women are often good at small talk but we're not always as good at listening. We have two ears and one mouth for a reason, so try to practise using them in this ratio if you have a tendency to take over.

BAD HABITS

If you make a bad first impression then it can take 21 further interactions before you change the other person's perception of you. Most of us are not lucky enough to get the chance to meet with someone that many times so we need to get it right first time.

A person, meeting you for the first time, may not remember what you have said but they will remember any bad habits you have up to 3 months later. This can mean anything from leaving your mobile switched on, constantly flicking your hair, smoking, swearing, drumming your fingers, wearing jangly jewellery, having dirty fingernails and so on. To be really sure about your habits check with your friends. Make sure you don't do something they daren't mention to you.

COMFORT

Last but not least, make sure your attire is comfortable. There is nothing worse than watching someone constantly pulling at the hem of their skirt, or adjusting their belt.

Test your shoes too. Blistered heels will not create the impact you wished for.

Always try on your outfit at least once before wearing it. Make sure the fit is correct and you feel great in it. It will be less for you to worry about on the day so you can get on with the job at hand.

Excuses, Excuses

"In think I was born never wanting to grow up."
Mary Quant - Fashion Designer

It's so easy, when you get older, to make excuses about the way you look. At the end of the day though this is just a cop out.

My mother-in-law, Audrey, is in her 80s. In the summertime she walks to the local lido and swims every day. Her garden is her passion. Not only does it look magnificent but it has the added advantage of keeping her physically in shape. She is not afraid to take holidays on her own and will never be short of someone to talk to. She has always had a sense of style, and reaching her ninth decade has done nothing to alter that view. A long time wearer of skirts and dresses, she took the plunge a couple of years ago and decided to try out trousers for the first time. A new addition to her wardrobe has now made itself known. She even purchased a pair of jeans – so who says you can be too old to wear those? In her wisdom, she realises the benefits of getting the foundation right. The result – her body looks as shapely today as it did when she was much younger.

If a lady of 80 plus has the wherewithal to care about her appearance then so should you. So no more excuses!

Here is a list of the excuses I hear on a regular basis, along with my answers. I hope you find them helpful.

It's not worth dressing up as I have small children and their dirty hands get everywhere.

The answer to this one is to wear garments with a pattern. This way the dirt is less likely to show up. If you're still taking the children to school then a coat with a pattern is a great way to look modern without looking mucky and unkempt. Team it with dark denim jeans and funky trainers so it becomes practical as well.

My teenage daughter thinks I'm too old to wear modern clothes, so I now live in my tracksuit.

This statement could well say more about your daughter than it does about you. Imagine yourself at her age. How would you feel if your mum was wearing clothes the same as yours? The key is to adapt the trends. If your daughter wears skinny jeans with cropped tops and high heels then wear yours with a boot cut to flatter the legs and team with a cashmere sweater. You can add a belt or a stunning piece of jewellery. That way you're still modern but adding your own spin to it makes it more suitable for your age.

I don't want to be noticed, so I tend to stick to clothes that cover me up.

Whether you like it or not, you *will* be noticed. It's better to be noticed for the right reasons than the wrong ones. Understated clothes can still be stylish. Baggy, shapeless clothes that shroud your body cannot. So choose clothes that are not fussy, in fabrics and colours that suit you. Let others notice how lovely you look rather than be seen hiding away in a corner.

I feel really fat so I'll change my image when I lose the weight.

When you've lost the weight – what are you hoping for? If the answer is to feel confident and look fantastic then why put it off until some future date in time? Select garments that will flatter your body shape and colouring now. You'll instantly look and feel so much better. The compliments will flow and others may think you've lost weight already. Getting the foundation garments right is another step you can take. A well-fitted bra can knock off up to a stone.

Wearing pattern in the correct scale can also disguise any lumps and bumps.

I never have any money to spend on myself. All my money goes on my family.

When I hear this, the emergency procedures on an aircraft come to mind. In the case of a potential crash, adults are advised to put on their life jackets and take the oxygen masks before they attend to their children. The premise being that if the adult dies, the children cannot take care of themselves so they too will die. I feel the same way about taking care of your appearance. Do you want your child's role model to be a mum who sacrifices everything; consequently looking dowdy and frumpy? Would you want them to do that for their children? Or would you prefer them to have a healthy belief that mum takes care of herself, looks terrific and of whom they're really proud?

Life is too short to worry about the way I look.

Life is short, there is no doubt about that, but the way you look can affect what happens to you in that lifetime. The impact you make and the confidence you have can all make your life easier to enjoy. Dressing to suit your personality and body shape is as easy, once you know how, as dressing in any old clothes. The difference in results? Enormous!

I don't like my legs, so I live in trousers and never really feel feminine.

Actually, I'm not a big fan of mine either – though my husband thinks they are my best feature! I too tend to like my trousers but if you team them with a sexy top, you can still look stunning. I do wear skirts and dresses too but with patterned tights and boots. This still looks youthful and I do actually feel very womanly. Shoes, of course, can make all the difference. Try walking around in a killer pair of shoes, preferably with a low front and high heel or wedge. Your legs will look amazing and you may change your mind about the way they look.

I don't have money to spare on new clothes.

Luckily for you, these days you don't need lots of money to look great. Designer labels are now creeping into high street stores – so you can buy good quality at a really reasonable price. Supermarkets sell cashmere sweaters at a third of the cost you would expect to pay in a specialist store. Spend any money you have on getting the basics right. A great coat, boots, a pair of trousers (or a skirt) and a great sweater are your essentials. If you have a large bust then make sure you don't skimp on buying the correct size bra. Tops and accessories can be picked up for very little cost. Choose wisely and you'll always look stunning.

I don't want to look like mutton dressed as lamb.

You won't if you follow the guidelines in this book. Don't make the mistake of wearing something you looked great in 20 years ago – it just won't work. Mini skirts, really low cut tops and 5 inch stilettos spring to mind. Look at the trends in the shops and adapt accordingly. Don't try and squeeze yourself into something that is too small. Sizes vary enormously according to manufacturer – even in the same store. Drop any ego and wear garments that flatter your shape rather than worry about what size is on the label. It is eminently possible to look youthful without looking ridiculous.

I'm too old to change.

You're never too old to do *anything*. These days you read about 70 year old women running marathons, giving birth, writing novels and other such marvellous achievements.

Age is a state of mind. You really are as old as you feel. A change of outfit may well enable you to put the zing back into your life. Move out of your comfort zone by taking small steps – a change of colour, a new piece of jewellery, a pair of great fitting trousers, a new hair style. Once you look in the mirror and see your fabulous reflection then you may want to change more than just your image.

I don't have a man around, so why bother?

This is the 21st Century! You don't have to have a man around to want to feel special about yourself and look fantastic. Wise up and smarten up. That attitude will certainly ensure no man comes looking for you anyway. Make the most of what you've got and you'll be turning them away.

Sue Donnelly

Out With The Old...

"You'd be surprised how much it costs to look this cheap!"

Dolly Parton, Singer, songwriter

As we get older it's only reasonable to expect that we've collected some baggage along the way. If the baggage has a high emotional content then it can be painful to deal with. It can also affect our future and how we deal with situations that arise and people we meet.

There is a widely held belief that if we de-clutter our lives of the things that are holding us back then we can create space to allow us to enjoy new and exciting experiences.

A similar idea lies behind a detox plan. The idea is to eliminate, over a short period of time, foods that are toxin related. The resulting benefits are a loss of weight, clearer skin, brighter mind and a more self confident you. But is this kind of treatment is geared only towards what we eat? What if we took the same

133

type of approach to the clothes that hang in our wardrobes? Wouldn't it be fabulous if a fashion detox could give us similar results?

The older we get, the more we tend to get stuck in a fashion rut. Black suits us. Baggy feels good on us. Those faithful old flatties never let you down. Added to which, have you ever noticed that however big your wardrobe is, the clothes you pick out from it daily only ever seem to shrink?

As we get older, our confidence around what to wear can also shrink. None of us want to look like mutton dressed as lamb, but we don't want to look like our grandmothers either. High Street stores tend to concentrate on either 18 year olds or senior citizens. As we fit into neither camp, it's easy to see why we get confused.

So if any of this rings true for you then try out the following and get ready for some fantastic compliments. If you can't do this today then make sure you find some time to do it SOON. This is important so please don't procrastinate.

Step One: Sort out your wardrobe

The following three steps will make sure you only have garments that make you feel wonderful. Just like a detox plan, it's about replacing things that make you look and feel low with those that will energise and brighten your whole being. Don't stop at clothes though, remember your jewellery, shoes and makeup can also benefit from this treatment plan.

If you haven't worn something in two years then throw it out. There is always a good reason why it's still hanging there and not being worn.

Be ruthless. If it's too small then don't make the mistake of keeping it until you've lost weight. It will act as a constant reminder that you are now a larger size. Instead, prepare to celebrate any future weight loss by buying something new when you've succeeded.

Get rid of mistakes. If it doesn't make you look (or feel) great, if you're tired of it or if it still has its tags then return it, sell it to a clothes agency, give it to charity or give it to a friend – if it will suit her.

If it has a great deal of sentimentality linked to it but you never wear it then put it in a box, and tuck it under your bed or in the basement. But don't let it take up valuable space in your closet if you don't wear it on a weekly basis. Look at it again in 6 months and see how you feel about it then. If you feel the same then keep it hidden away. Repeat at regular intervals until you're ready to let it go. Ask yourself why it's so important to keep hold of. What does it make you think or feel that you don't have now? What's missing from your life?

Make repairs. This can also include dying it, if it's the wrong colour, altering the hemline, taking it in at the seams, changing the buttons and so on. If you don't take it to be repaired in one month then you know you're really not that crazy about it – so throw it out.

The comfort factor. Comfy old clothes are okay for slobbing about the house and chilling out but when it comes to the outside world, comfort does not replace style. Clothes should always make the most of your figure and there's no reason why you can't combine style *and* comfort.

There are certain items that must go – whether or not they fit and whether or not you think they suit you. For example – high waisted, tapered trousers with pleats, mini skirts, jackets with huge shoulder pads and any garment that would look better on your mother needs to go!

On the whole, if you haven't worn something in two years, it needs to go but there are exceptions. If you're still madly in love with an older garment, that has worn well, is still stylish and makes you feel special then keep it.

Step Two: Organise the garments into separate piles

1. Looks good and fits – or would if it was repaired.

2. Would look great if it fit.

3. Never looked that great but is almost new.

4. Hasn't been worn for over 2 years.

Step Three: Keep the first category and get rid of the others

Clothes for the 'no mercy' pile – for example: tartan, kilts, anything flannel, especially shirts and certain nightgowns, Logo tee shirts, nylon tracksuits, tapered trousers.

Remember, you can make money by selling "as new" clothes to a clothing agency. Alternatively, if it has a designer label then you could try selling it on ebay.

You may already find that a great weight has been lifted psychologically. You'll have less stuff to store and sort through and clearing out clutter is very liberating. To make way for the new you have to clear out the old. It will do you no favours to hang onto things you no longer need.

Clothes are all about providing the wearer with confidence. A well–tailored, classic garment, such as a coat, can remain current over a period of 3+ years. 'Fashionable' items should be worn for the season only. That's why it's never worth spending too much money on them.

Fashion items that will stand the test of time are:

- A single-breasted jacket

- A classic winter coat

- An A Line skirt

- A cashmere sweater

- A trendy belt

- Wide legged masculine trousers

- A well cut T-shirt or two

- Jeans that fit perfectly

- A great bag

- A pair of knee length or ankle boots

**Items that will add 10 years to your age
AND NEED TO GO!**

- Any 'fashion' item that has just come round for a second time

- High waisted, tapered trousers with pleats. BURN them – they will make you look short legged, big bummed and bulky round the tummy!

- Shoulder pads in anything

- Big, baggy Tee-shirts with short sleeves

- Shapeless cotton shift dresses with a round neckline and no sleeves – especially if patterned

- Leggings – even if you have legs like Elle Macpherson

- Ankle length pop socks

- Tapered jeans – especially in stone wash denim

- Mini skirts

- Leather trousers – unforgiving!

Once you've de-cluttered then bear the following in mind...'

AIR YOUR CLOTHING

Install a hook on the outside of the door. Use it to air out the clothing you've worn before returning it to the closet. Doing this will save you money on dry cleaning. Excessive dry cleaning can ruin a garment – so only get it dry cleaned if the item is soiled.

USE A FULL LENGTH MIRROR

Install one on the inside of the closet door or use a free standing mirror. You need to see your clothing in its entirety to see if an item is really working for you.

LET THERE BE LIGHT

It is absolutely essential to have a bright light installed in your closet. You need to see what you have in order to wear it.

STAY ORGANISED

To manage your new collection (and to make it easier to combine your existing garments) hang clothes by type. Put your jackets together, your trousers, tops and so on. You'll be amazed how many different combinations you can find. If you prefer then you can also differentiate by colour. Do the same for your boots, shoes and sandals. This should save you time when dressing.

STORAGE

Avoid wire coat hangers as the can ruin the shape of your garments. Buy wood (cedar is best) or wider plastic hangers instead.

Knits should be folded rather than hung on hangers, otherwise they may stretch.

Tailored pieces need padded or wood hangers.

Trousers and skirts should be hung from the waist with clip hangers. If trousers are creased then try hanging them upside down from the hems or invest in a trouser press.

If you are short of space then pack away last season's clothes. Garments should be placed in a dark, dry and well-ventilated part of your home. They need to be protected from insects, dirt and odour.

TAKE CARE OF YOUR SHOES

Take your favourite shoes to be re-heeled and resoled. Get rid of outdated shoes. Nothing can date an outfit faster. Toss any shoe that is uncomfortable. Realize that over the years, your shoe size has changed. Your foot has gotten bigger or wider and it's not going to shrink! Invest in shoe trees or keep shoes in shoeboxes. Stuff shoes with tissue or newspaper to hold their shape. Take a picture of the shoe and staple it on the box so that you won't have to open *every* box to find your shoes.

BAGS

If you have spent lots of money on a fabulous bag then make sure you keep it in the cloth bag in which it came. If you aren't using it for a while then stuff it with tissue paper to keep its shape intact.

MAKE A LIST OF ANY 'GAPS'

Last but not least, take a good look at the garments you have chosen to keep. What is missing? Make a list of essential items such as a jacket or skirt. When you next go shopping, take the list with you and ONLY buy what is on the list – NOTHING MORE!

Take a leaf out of the chic Parisienne's book. They always look stylish because they plan their wardrobe, and their shopping. So instead of buying individual garments on a whim, think about what they will complement in your existing collection. As a rule of thumb, if it doesn't go with three other items, don't buy it.

Treat yourself to a glass of something – you deserve it!

The Wise Woman Within

"The only real elegance is in the mind. If you've got that, the rest really follows from it."

Diana Vreeland - Fashion Journalist

Many of us, as we get older, are reluctant to look more modern, for a number of reasons:

- We are scared to shop in places like Top Shop or H&M, as we feel too old. Worse still, we don't want to wear what our daughters are wearing (and vice versa).

- Life begins at 40 but it can also be scary. Many of us feel like we've lost our identity. What are we supposed to look like at 40 or 50?

- To be thought of as "mutton dressed as lamb" is horrifying!

- We feel that we look older so we wear an older person's clothes.

- We believe that chic, classic tailoring will see us through. Sometimes it will, but on the wrong person it can be very ageing – think 'power dressing', shoulder pads and scarves of the 80's.

- We are in a rut and don't know how to get out of it.

- It's easier not to bother.

If you fit into any (or all) of these categories then read on. Here are my top tips for the wise woman to look modern and stylish – whatever your age or shape.

ADAPT THE TRENDS

Look at what's in fashion in the magazines and high street stores but, instead of following slavishly, take the main idea and adapt to your own shape. Current trends (at the time of writing) feature nautical, safari and boho styles. A pair of pale trousers teamed with a striped or plain T-shirt and a single-breasted, fitted jacket will provide the nautical flavour. If you have an angular body then swap the jacket for a boxy denim one. Safari jackets don't suit everyone but a wrap dress in a jungle or animal print may look fantastic. Just don't overdo the accessories if the print is bold. A layered skirt and multi-coloured peasant top may be too much to carry off. Try an A-line skirt with a plain or patterned top and wear it with boots, wedges or flip-flops to get the same type of look. A pair of jeans teamed with a cashmere sweater will always look modern and stylish. Stick to boot cut for a more flattering effect. Skinny jeans are very unforgiving unless tucked into boots and worn with a longer top.

ACCESSORISE

Too many accessories can give you the "Christmas Tree" effect. When you get older, less is often more, especially if you are petite. Choose wisely and pick just one great accessory to add some dramatic impact. A large, ethnic necklace or bracelet, a leather linked belt slung low around the hips, a fur gilet, or a cropped cardigan (great if you're small chested) will all look fabulous.

Don't forget your hosiery either. We tend to think that tights are just mundane things we put on everyday. This year, they are making a statement of their own. So use flesh fishnets or dark patterned tights if you want to make a statement and still look good.

ENHANCE YOUR BODY

Understand what fabrics and shapes suit you best. Don't ignore it. Contoured shapes need fabrics that skim over the curves. Angular shapes need stiff, starchy fabrics to enhance the straight lines. Make the most of your assets – you now know what they are – and show them off to dazzling effect.

BE TRUE TO YOUR PERSONALITY

Be authentic in your dress. There is nothing more draining than trying to be someone else.

WEAR THE CORRECT SIZE

There is no actual standardisation in the size of women's clothing in the UK, so all of us will have at least 3 different sizes in our wardrobe, and that's not counting garments for fat/thin days! If you wear clothes that are too small then you will look bigger. If you wear clothes that are too big, you'll look drowned!

WEAR FLATTERING COLOURS

Especially near to your face. Warm skins need warm tones like olives, golds and browns to enhance your glow. Cool skins need cool tones like blue and pink to flatter your skin. The wrong colour can drain and add years.

FOUNDATION IS KEY

Wearing the right size underwear is critical. Get yourself measured – if it's been longer than a year. If your tum's got a life of its own then try magic knickers.

STAND UP STRAIGHT

A poor posture can ruin any outfit. So if you've made all this effort then make sure you can carry it off to your best advantage by standing tall. In yoga, they refer to the 'bandhas' and in pilates, the 'core' or 'powerhouse'. This is the place in your body where you need to concentrate your effort. Place 2 fingers widthways below your navel and pull it in. Make sure you can also breathe! If done regularly, it will strengthen your abdominals and make you appear leaner. Imagine a string being pulled from the top of your head. Move into this position and pull your shoulders down and back. There you have it – perfect posture and an instantly younger, thinner you.

EXPERIMENT

Don't be afraid to experiment. If you've had the same look for years then make the transition easier by adding small changes until you become comfortable and confident with the 'new look' you. Swap trousers for the occasional skirt and try a belt round your hips. If you are already adventurous then try more modern garments and see how you feel. You can always use mail order catalogues and try them on at home, where the mirrors don't lie. This also gives you the opportunity to combine any possible purchase with your existing garments.

SHOP WISELY

If you have read this book all the way through then you will know which items to spend money on and which can be purchased cheaply. You are now aware of the staples that make up your wardrobe so you can add to your basics rather than buying a garment that doesn't go with anything else. Always take a shopping list and don't detract from it. Think in terms of outfits and not garments. Only go to sales if you know for sure that there is something worth buying. Otherwise give them a miss. After all, it is only stock that the shop no longer wants and there's *always* a reason for that.

USE THE ART OF DISGUISE

If you're feeling under the weather then use the tricks of the trade. Use large spectacles or sunglasses to hide dark circles or puffiness around the eyes, wear a flattering colour around your face, divert attention by clever use of jewellery, apply your favourite lipstick and cheer yourself up with a spray of a fabulous fragrance.

LOVE YOUR LOOK AND LIVE YOUR LIFE

Be proud of what you have achieved. Live your life with passion and zest for all things – not just your clothes. Dressing well is just the first step on the road to confidence and success. Enjoy each day and make the most of every opportunity that comes your way. Celebrate your age, pamper yourself, learn to accept the inevitable compliments – as you'll be receiving lots of them from now on – and be radiant in your magnificence.

As Christian Dior once said: "Zest is the secret of all beauty. There is no beauty that is attractive without zest."

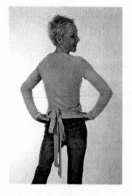

Accentuate – the accent on U, your image and your impact.

Sue Donnelly is an Image Coach with a wide experience of working with people, both in a corporate environment and on a personal basis. She has held a variety of management positions for Thomas Cook, Citibank and Insights Learning & Development where image and relationship building were crucial factors in attracting and retaining business partnerships. Sue's work with individuals enables them to find a style of dress that reflects their inner values and unique personality, elevating self-esteem and confidence. Corporate work includes personal branding seminars and workshops enabling consistency to be reinforced throughout an organisation. She has been featured in national magazines and newspapers, writes a style column for Health Plus magazine, and has been invited to appear on prime time television. She is also the style expert for www.expertsonline.tv and a volunteer for the breast cancer charity, Look Good Feel Better. A qualified life coach, fitness instructor and workshop facilitator with the skills and the passion to help men and women look and feel good about themselves in an authentic way, whatever their age or shape. Her previous books, *The 80/20 Makeover* and *"Does My Belly Look Big In This?"*,,are also available from www.bookshaker.com

To contact Sue...
Phone: 0845 123 5107
Website: www.accentuate.me.uk

THE 80/20 MAKEOVER

- **Women: Buy Clothes You Actually Wear**

- **Men: Spend Less Time Wandering Round Shops**

- **Discover Your Body Shape Then Cheat Nature**

- **Find & Use The Colours That Make You Glow**

SUE DONNELLY

www.bookshaker.com

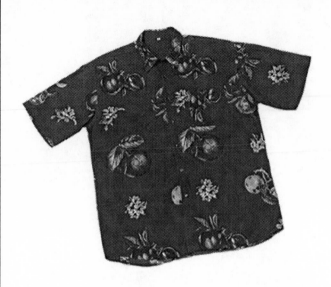

Does my belly look big in this?

look big in this?

a common sense style guide for
men who care what they wear

SUE DONNELLY

www.bookshaker.com

Printed in the United Kingdom
by Lightning Source UK Ltd.
125668UK00001B/133/A